THE
PROBIOTIC KITCHEN

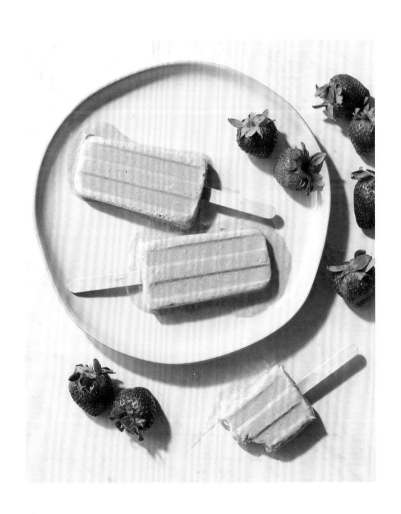

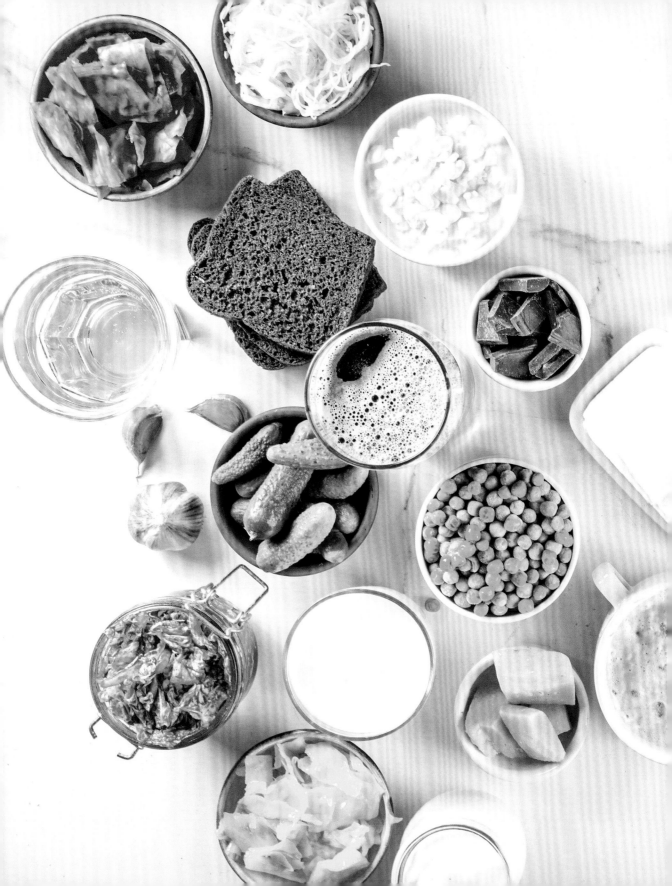

THE
PROBIOTIC KITCHEN

More Than 100 Delectable, Natural, and

Supplement-Free Probiotic and Prebiotic Recipes

KELLI FOSTER

HARVARD
COMMON
PRESS

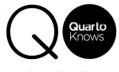

Inspiring | Educating | Creating | Entertaining

Brimming with creative inspiration, how-to projects, and useful information to enrich your everyday life, Quarto Knows is a favorite destination for those pursuing their interests and passions. Visit our site and dig deeper with our books into your area of interest: Quarto Creates, Quarto Cooks, Quarto Homes, Quarto Lives, Quarto Drives, Quarto Explores, Quarto Gifts, or Quarto Kids.

First Published in 2020 by The Harvard Common Press, an imprint of The Quarto Group,
100 Cummings Center, Suite 265-D, Beverly, MA 01915, USA.
T (978) 282-9590 F (978) 283-2742 QuartoKnows.com

The Harvard Common Press titles are also available at discount for retail, wholesale, promotional, and bulk purchase. For details, contact the Special Sales Manager by email at specialsales@quarto.com or by mail at The Quarto Group, Attn: Special Sales Manager, 100 Cummings Center, Suite 265-D, Beverly, MA 01915, USA.

24 23 22 21 20   1 2 3 4 5

ISBN: 978-1-55832-989-8

Digital edition published in 2020
eISBN: 978-1-55832-990-4

Library of Congress Cataloging-in-Publication Data

Names: Foster, Kelli C., author.
Title: The probiotic kitchen : more than 100 delectable, natural, and
  supplement-free probiotic and prebiotic recipes / Kelli Foster.
Description: Beverly, MA : Harvard Common Press, 2020. | Includes index.
Identifiers: LCCN 2019033070 (print) | LCCN 2019033071 (ebook) | ISBN
  9781558329898 (trade paperback) | ISBN 9781558329904 (eISBN)
Subjects: LCSH: Digestive organs--Diseases--Diet therapy--Recipes. |
  Probiotics--Popular works. | Prebiotics--Popular works. | Colitis--Diet
  therapy--Recipes. | Candidiasis--Diet therapy--Recipes. | Food
  allergy--Diet therapy--Recipes. | LCGFT: Cookbooks.
Classification: LCC RC806 .F67 2020 (print) | LCC RC806 (ebook) | DDC
  641.5/63--dc23
LC record available at https://lccn.loc.gov/2019033070
LC ebook record available at https://lccn.loc.gov/2019033071

Design and Layout: Laura Klynstra
Cover Image: Maria Siriano
Photography: Maria Siriano, except for pages 2-3, 7, 13-45, 62-63, 74, 85-87, 102-103, 118-119, 136-137, 155, 166-167, 175-181, 186, 193, 197

Printed in China

The information in this book is for educational purposes only. It is not intended to replace the advice of a physician or medical practitioner. Please see your health-care provider before beginning any new health program.

For Owen

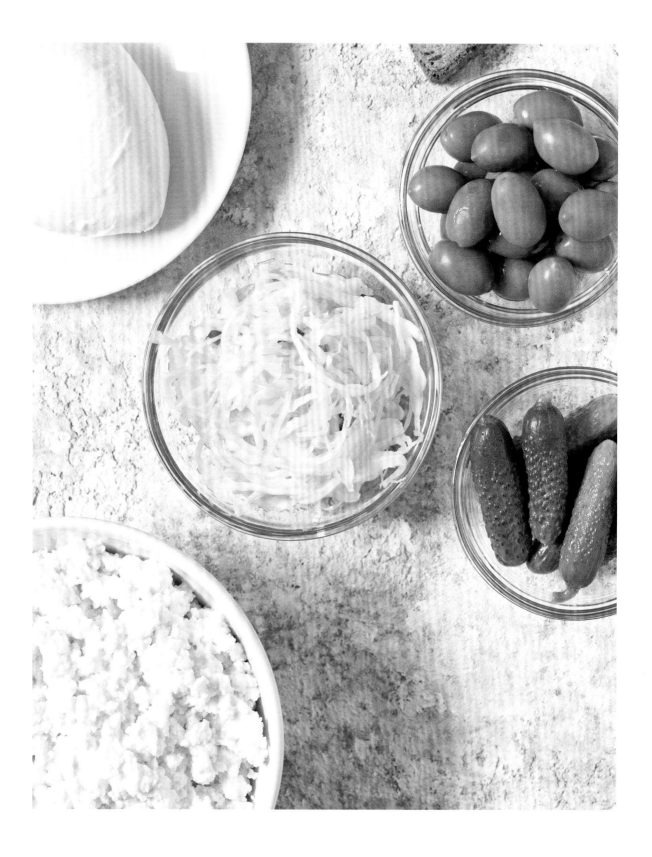

Contents

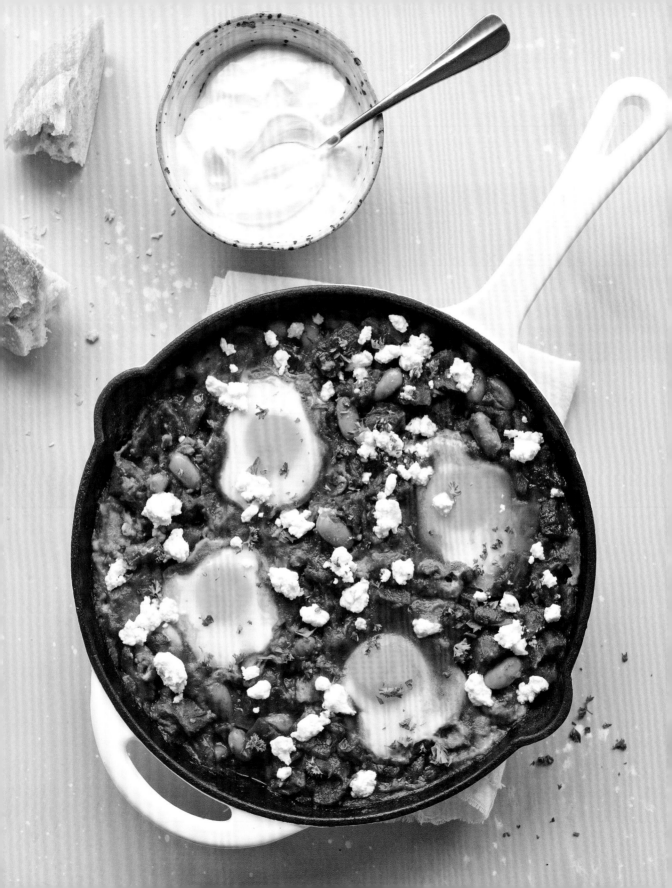

The Probiotic Life

Recently, as I ate a Buddha bowl for lunch, thrown together with a mess of ingredients in an effort to clean out my fridge at the end of the week, I noticed that nearly all the ingredients—miso paste, scallions, avocado, fermented vegetables, and Greek yogurt—contained either probiotics or prebiotics. For the first time, it dawned on me that I've been unintentionally (but regularly) including these gut-friendly foods in my diet, long before I knew about the benefits of probiotics and before I even knew that prebiotics were something to know about. I realized that, beyond the Buddha bowls I frequently eat for lunch or dinner, between yogurt bowls, smoothies, sauces, dressings, snacks, and fermented kraut I add to just about everything, I was incorporating a variety of natural probiotic foods into my diet pretty consistently. Turns out it was easy, and I wasn't launching into any DIY home fermenting projects or taking supplements to add more probiotics to my diet.

And you know what? There's a good chance the same is true for you.

The reason I'm so sure is simple. It's because probiotics (and prebiotics) are a natural component of so many common and readily available foods and even drinks. Sure, there are supplements aplenty these days, but they are far from the only way to get your probiotics. There is such an array of wholesome foods to choose from at your local grocer or farmers market that already come loaded with probiotic benefits. And better yet, there are so many interesting and delicious ways to easily work these probiotic foods into your diet as meals and snacks.

This cookbook is all about showing you just how easy it is to incorporate naturally probiotic-rich foods into your everyday diet. And, like I said, you may already be eating them without even knowing it, which puts you one step ahead of the game! The heart and soul of this book centers around widely available foods that contain probiotics and prebiotics made into more than a hundred approachable, healthy recipes to turn the natural probiotic foods you purchase, like yogurt, kimchi, and miso paste, into meals from breakfast through dinner and even dessert.

Let's get started!

What Are Probiotics and What Do They Do for You?

Without getting too much into the science (because we're all eager to get cooking), probiotics are living microorganisms—sometimes referred to as "good" bacteria—that have health benefits, particularly in maintaining a healthy gut and digestive system. (Certain types of yeasts, which are not bacteria, also deliver probiotic benefits.)

That's right, not all bacteria (also known as "gut flora" in the digestive system) are bad. Probiotics work to rebalance the good bacteria in your gut, keeping the bad bacteria in check and thus contributing to your digestive health.

Probiotics have been touted for doing everything from maintaining and improving digestive function to helping cure digestive ailments, offering immune benefits, reducing inflammation, and so much more. And while there's been extensive research recently into all the many ways probiotics can improve our overall health and a long list of benefits they can offer, it seems we've only just scratched the surface—there's still a lot of research left to be done. But one thing we know for sure, which I've experienced firsthand, is that probiotics help to maintain good digestive health.

Not only do you want to eat more foods that contain natural probiotics, but it's important to eat a variety of these foods. There are various classifications of probiotics, and they're not all created equal. Different species and strains offer different potential benefits, so to make sure you're taking advantage of many of these benefits, rather than just one or two, it's helpful to introduce an array of natural gut-friendly foods to your diet. That's what this book is for.

What Probiotics Will Not Do for You

While probiotics come with a host of health benefits, they are by no means a cure-all or a one-size-fits-all solution. You are also not likely to see their benefits instantaneously or from a single use. This is a marathon, not a sprint, and to really feel the good effects of ingesting probiotics, you want to gradually make them a regular part of your diet.

The exact benefits of probiotics can also vary from person to person. Think of your gut flora as an internal fingerprint. Everyone's is different, and yours is totally unique to you, so probiotics can have different effects for different people. Because our gut flora aren't identical, each of us is likely to experience a slight variation in the benefits of probiotics and how quickly we see them.

Remember, research around probiotics is still in the early days as far as learning all the ways probiotics will have an impact on our overall health and wellness.

Probiotics Naturally: All the Foods That Are Probiotic

Eating natural probiotic foods is far from a new trend. Probiotics are naturally found in all different foods, and cultures around the world have been consuming probiotic-rich fermented foods for thousands of years.

My favorite way to incorporate probiotics into my daily routine is with wholesome real foods, both because it feels the most natural and because it's extremely easy. While it's true that dietary supplements will give you the highest dose of probiotics, there is also a variety of nutritious foods—such as kefir, kombucha, miso paste, tempeh, and yogurt, to name a few—that contain natural probiotics, among a host of other healthful benefits.

Chances are you're already eating some of them and didn't know they were probiotic. To be sure you're at the top of your gut-health game, read the label with the list of ingredients on natural probiotic foods. You're on the lookout for the term *live active cultures* (or *live and active cultures*). This is your cue that a food contains probiotics and that cultures were added *after* pasteurization. You might even see a list of the cultures that are included right there on the label. There are some foods, particularly dairy items, that are pasteurized after the cultures are added, thus killing off the bacteria and the gut-health benefits.

While you will find a great selection of naturally probiotic-rich foods at grocery and health food stores, another good place to source them is at farmers markets. There you'll find small-batch producers with interesting items, including different types of fermented kraut and vegetables, local yogurts and kefir, and perhaps even cheese, that you're not as likely to find from commercial brands. In chapter 1, we'll take a walk though the most common foods that naturally contain probiotics, which will serve as a great primer for the recipes ahead.

Don't Forget the Prebiotics! Why You Need Them and Where to Find Them

I briefly mentioned prebiotics earlier, and that's because we can't possibly talk about probiotics without discussing prebiotics. The two work hand in hand, and each plays an important role in maintaining gut health.

In short, prebiotics are food for probiotics. They're nondigestible ingredients that nourish good gut bacteria and enable them to flourish and thrive, which ultimately benefits our overall health and well-being.

While prebiotic supplements are available, as are probiotics, perhaps the easiest way to get your fill is with the long list of foods that already have them, such as avocados, bananas, raw asparagus, scallions, onions, garlic, whole oats, and barley. As with probiotics, you can certainly eat natural prebiotic foods on their own, but this duo is even more powerful when you eat them together. For that reason, you'll see plenty of recipes throughout the book that include both probiotics and prebiotics. We'll take a closer look at common prebiotic foods in chapter 1.

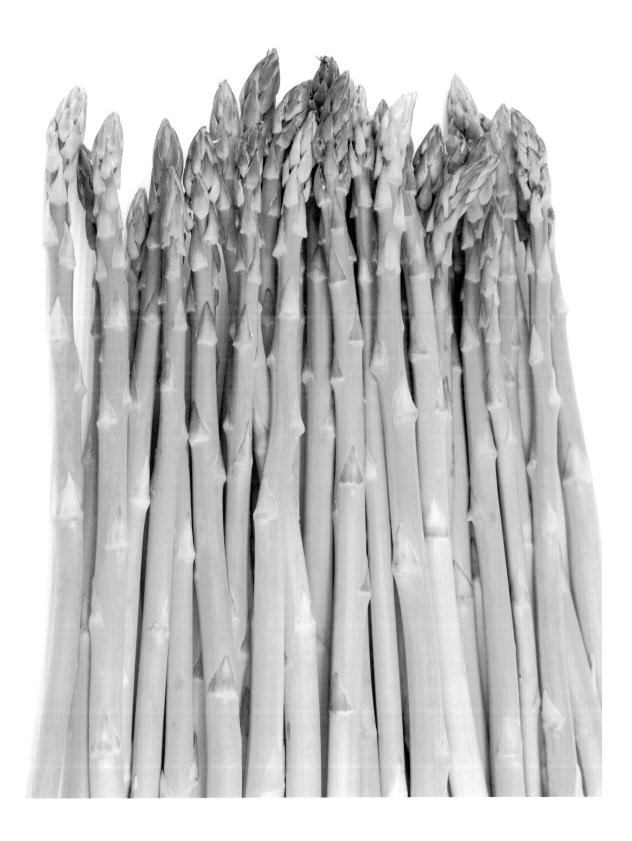

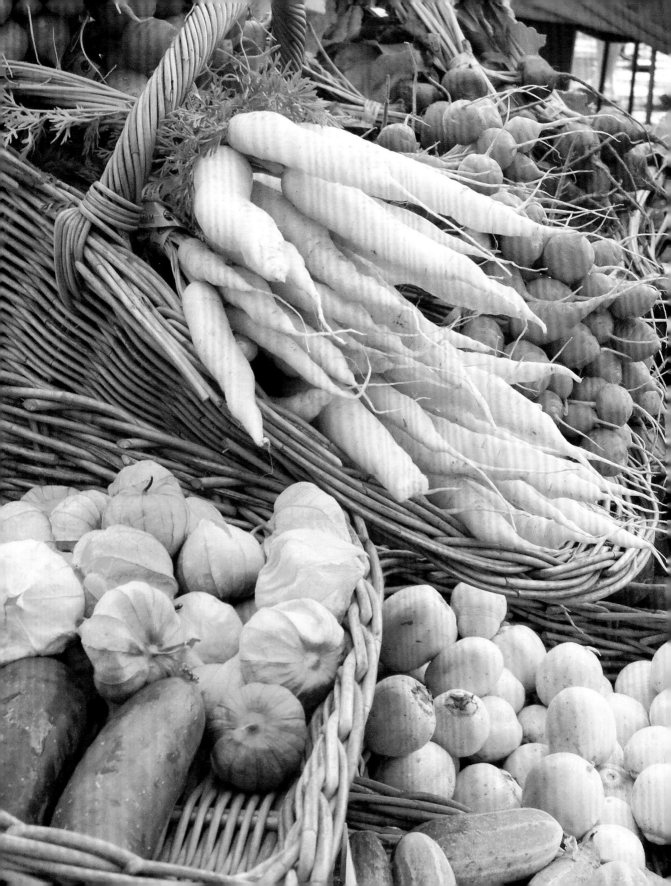

Sourcing Probiotics 1: Buying Your Own

A Shopper's Guide to Probiotic and Prebiotic Foods

Good news: You don't have to take up home fermentation or load up on supplements to treat your body to more probiotics. In fact, I believe the absolute easiest way to eat more probiotics on a regular basis starts in the aisles of your local market. That includes everywhere from health food stores and Whole Foods to big-name grocers and farmers markets.

Farmers markets are a particular favorite for sourcing small-batch fermented foods and drinks, as well as other probiotic and prebiotic foods. In addition to supporting local small businesses and knowing where my food comes from, I can be sure that these items are often minimally treated, organic, and extremely fresh.

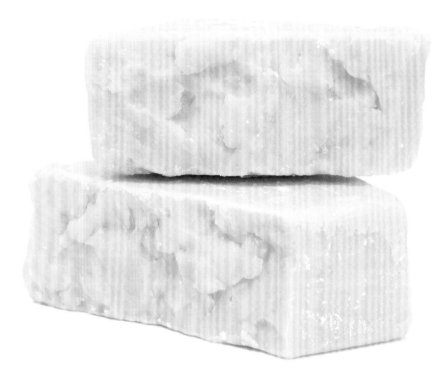

PROBIOTIC FOODS

Aged Cheese

While most types of cheese are fermented, not all contain probiotics, so you'll need to take a close look at the label. Raw, unpasteurized aged cheese is where you'll find the most benefit, though the number of probiotics found in cheese is limited. The most common types of cheese boasting probiotic benefits are aged Gouda, aged cheddar, aged mozzarella, and some varieties of aged Gruyère. You may also find probiotics in some raw and unpasteurized soft cheeses.

Probiotic Coconut Yogurt

This probiotic powerhouse is for the serious coconut lover. Not only is the nondairy yogurt an option for those avoiding lactose and a great source of probiotics, it also has an irresistibly thick, rich texture that makes it a real treat. Look for brands like Anita's, The Coconut Cult, COYO, and GT's Living Foods.

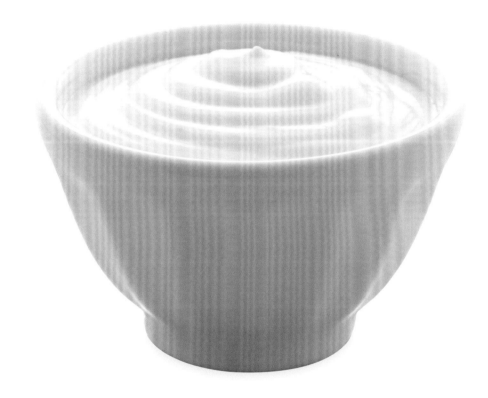

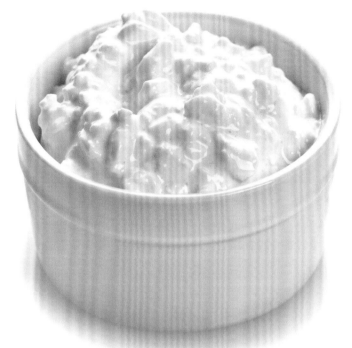

Cultured Cottage Cheese

Cultured cottage cheese has the same creamy texture, curds, and slightly tangy taste as regular cottage cheese and it can be used in all the same ways. What sets it apart is that it's made with live-active cultures and boasts ample probiotic benefits. Be sure to check the label when buying cottage cheese to make sure you are getting the cultured variety, from brands such as Good Culture, Horizon Organic, or Nancy's.

Kefir

This delicious, fermented milk drink made from cow's or goat's milk and kefir grains has been around for thousands of years. The taste might remind you of yogurt, but unlike yogurt, it contains more strains of bacteria and is cultured longer, leaving it with even more probiotic benefits. Stick with plain, unsweetened milk kefir and avoid flavored kefir, which can be loaded with added sugar.

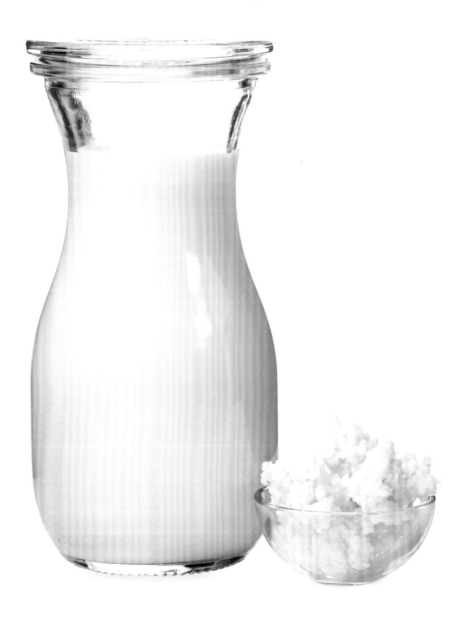

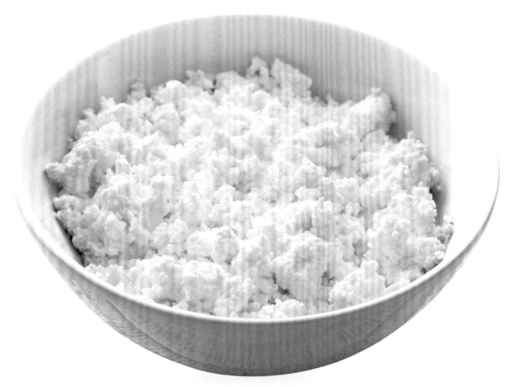

Cultured Farmer Cheese

This mild-mannered, cultured soft cheese has a spreadable texture and a taste that falls somewhere between ricotta and cottage cheese, although it is also slightly drier since most of the moisture has been pressed out. It can be used in both sweet and savory dishes. Look for brands such as Lifeway.

Kimchi

Kimchi is a traditional Korean side dish, packed with a mix of zesty, spicy flavors. Not only is it probiotically rich and great for gut health, but as a cabbage-based dish, it is also a good source of antioxidants and vitamins A, B, and C.

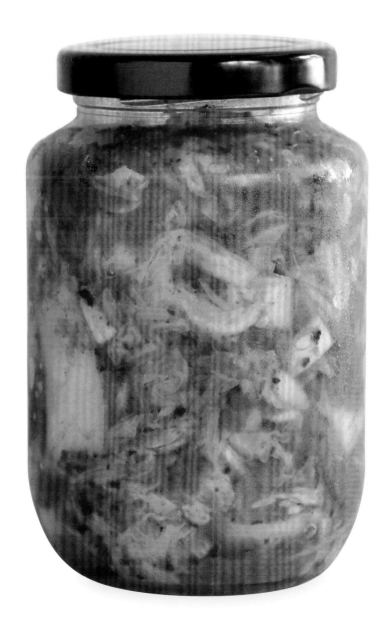

Kombucha

Kombucha is a fermented drink with a sour, fizzy taste that's rich in probiotics and antioxidants. It's made with either black or green tea, sugar, and yeast, and in addition to drinking it as is, there are many other fun ways to turn kombucha into different drinks, even condiments and desserts. You'll want to look at the label and choose options with no added sugar for the best health benefits.

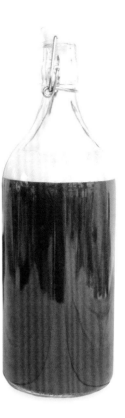

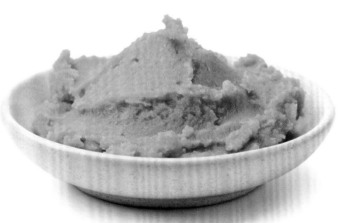

Miso Paste

Made from fermented soybeans, miso paste is a mainstay in Japanese cooking. It has a savory, nutty, umami-rich flavor, and adding a spoonful or two to soups, dressings, spreads, and even sweet dishes offers an instant boost of probiotics.

Pickles

Yes, even sour, fermented pickles contain probiotics. It's important to remember, though, that not all pickles are made through the process of fermentation. Those shelf-stable varieties found near the canned goods are pasteurized, and the cucumbers are pickled rather than fermented, meaning they don't contain probiotics. Choose fermented pickles from the refrigerated section of your grocer and remember to always read the label, checking the ingredient list for live active cultures.

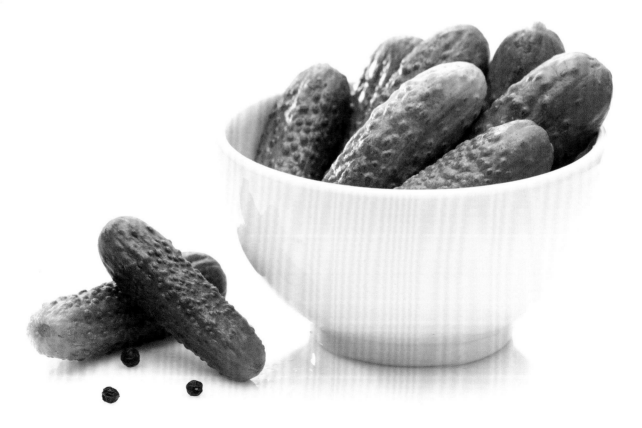

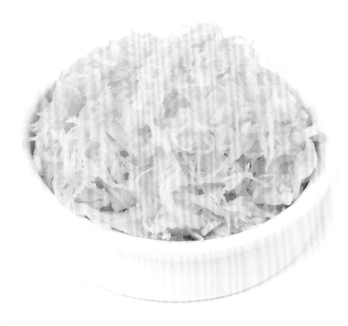

Sauerkraut

Gut-friendly sauerkraut is near the top of the list of foods naturally loaded with pro-biotics. While it's traditionally made with green cabbage, these days you'll find kraut made from an array of vegetables and aromatics, including red cabbage, beets, carrots, radishes, scallions, jalapeños, turmeric, and ginger.

Skip the sauerkraut in the canned-foods aisle, which is pasteurized and doesn't contain probiotics. Instead, choose fermented kraut from the refrigerated section of your grocer or from your local farmers market and look for the mention of live active cultures on the label.

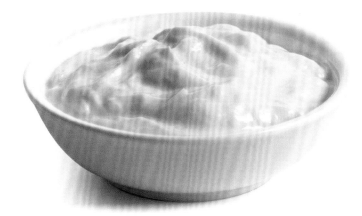

Skyr

Hailing from Iceland and now readily found in the United States, skyr is a fermented cheese product made from nonfat milk. But don't let that cheese-like description fool you; skyr is most like Greek yogurt, with a thicker, creamier texture, less tangy taste, and slightly higher amount of protein. It can be used in all the same ways you'd use yogurt, and the two can be used interchangeably in recipes.

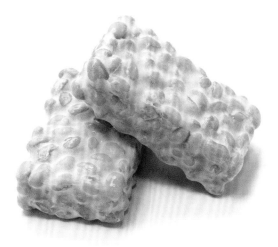

Tempeh

Probiotics aren't the only thing this popular high-protein meat alternative has going for it. Tempeh also delivers a long list of vitamins and minerals, including calcium, iron, and magnesium. Tempeh is made from fermented soybeans and takes the shape of a cake or patty, with a firm texture and nutty, savory flavor, that can be eaten raw, seared, sautéed, or baked.

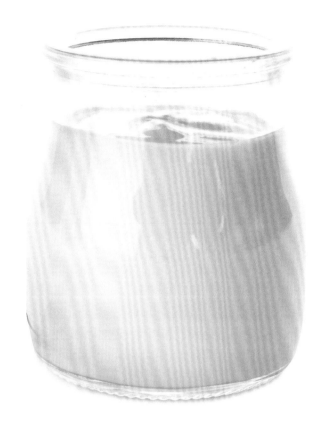

Yogurt

Yogurt, both regular and Greek, is one of the most common sources of probiotics. But here's the catch—while most yogurts fit the bill, not all yogurts contain probiotics. Check the label to be sure it contains live active cultures. And to maximize the health benefit of yogurt, stick with plain, unsweetened varieties, avoiding those bogged down with added sugar, which lessens the benefits of probiotics.

PREBIOTIC FOODS

Prebiotics act as food for probiotics and are an essential factor in enabling good bacteria to flourish in our digestive system. And just like probiotics, there is a wide variety of foods that naturally contain prebiotics. One of the first things to notice about this list is that many of these foods are also easy to find in your grocery store.

Alliums (cooked): Garlic, onions
Alliums (raw): Garlic, leeks, onions, and scallions
Asparagus (raw)
Avocado
Banana
Barley
Flaxseeds
Greens (raw): Dandelion greens, endive, frisee, and radicchio
Honey (raw)
Jerusalem artichoke
Jicama root
Legumes: Chickpeas, red kidney beans, lentils, and peas
Wheat bran
Whole oats

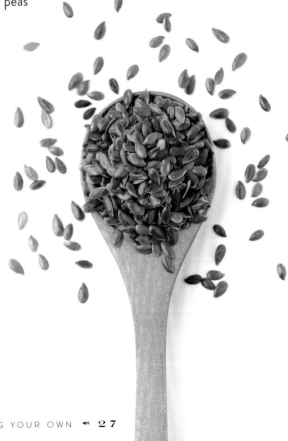

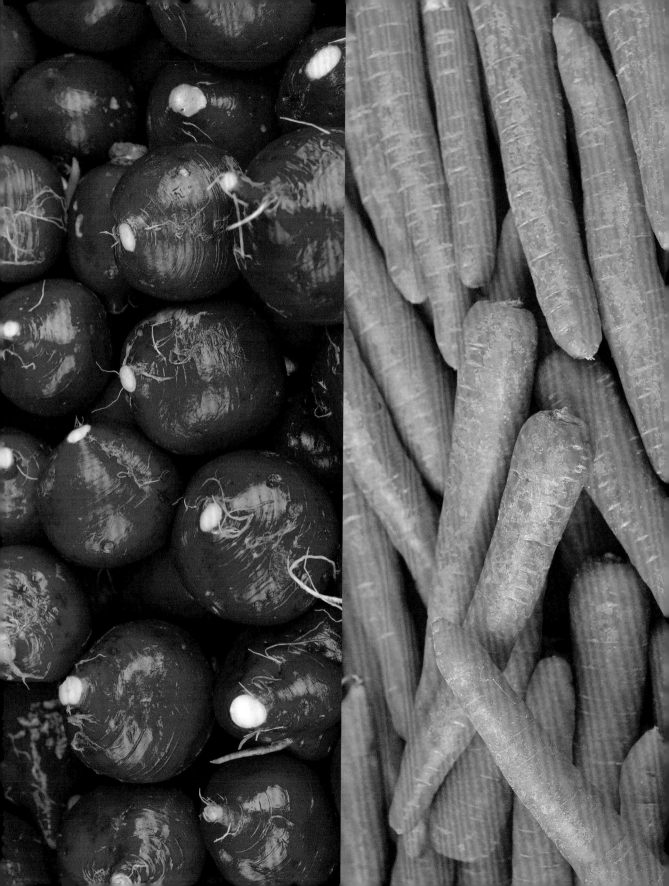

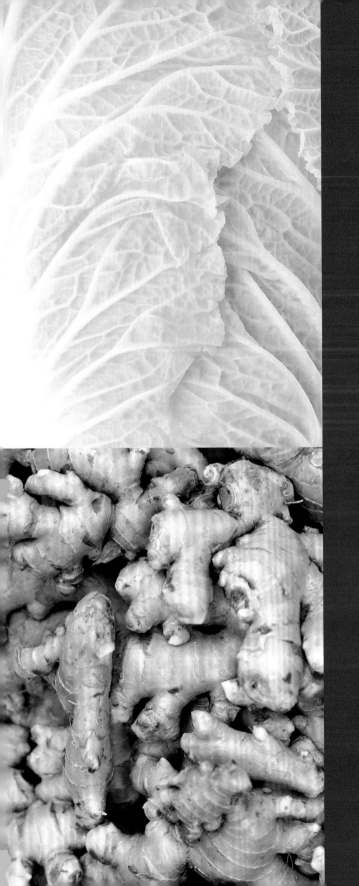

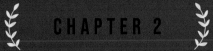

CHAPTER 2

Sourcing Probiotics 2: Making Your Own

A Primer on Fermentation: Easy DIY Ferments for Probiotics

Buying probiotic-rich foods is certainly convenient, but it's also just one way to get more probiotics in your diet. You can also do it yourself, including making your own yogurt or kefir, sauerkraut, kimchi, kombucha, fermented salsa and pickles, and so much more.

If you're a DIY-er who loves a good project, you'd probably enjoy home fermentation. You can make many of these foods at home. And even if you're not already a DIY-er, you've got this—trust me!

There are certain home fermentation projects that require a good deal of time, special equipment, and some precision, but there are many more that are easy to pull off. Sauerkraut, other vegetable krauts, tangy fermented vegetables, and even fermented salsa all fall under the latter category. If you've never fermented anything, these offer a great place to start. Not only are krauts and fermented vegetables surprisingly easy, versatile, and very forgiving, they don't require a whole lot of time or effort.

What Is Fermentation?

When it comes to home fermentation, one of the most common and easiest methods, and the one used in this book, is lacto-fermentation (or lactic acid fermentation). During the fermentation process, lactic acid bacteria consumes the sugars in the food, releasing lactic acid. This creates an acidic environment where only beneficial bacteria can survive.

Just about any vegetable can be fermented. You can alter the flavor of your ferments with aromatics, such as ginger and garlic, or a whole host of spices, including caraway seeds (popular in traditional sauerkraut), juniper berries, bay leaves, mustard seeds, coriander seeds, and turmeric, to name a few.

The DIY fermented vegetables in this chapter are all easy and super accessible to make. For each of them, there are essentially two steps: prepping and waiting. Each recipe starts by prepping the vegetables. Then, it's a matter of having some patience during the fermentation process and waiting until they have the flavor you enjoy. As for how many days you must wait, well, that can be the tricky part if you're just getting started because there isn't an exact amount of time or number of days. Fermented vegetables are ready to eat when they taste good to you. That can be two to three days if you prefer a mild flavor or up to a couple of weeks if you prefer a more intense flavor. You'll see exactly what I'm talking about once you give it a try. The number of probiotics will also increase the longer the vegetables are fermented. You'll know they're ready simply by tasting the vegetables every day (and yes, this is totally safe!).

Basic Small Batch Sauerkraut

If you're just getting started with home fermentation, sauerkraut is a really great place to begin. It is inexpensive, can be made in small batches, doesn't require a whole lot of gear, and, best of all, is surprisingly easy and nearly foolproof. Sauerkraut is made through the process of lacto-fermentation, and it involves just cabbage and salt.

Expect the process to take anywhere from three to fourteen days—it all depends on just how funky and flavorful you like your kraut. While the kraut will be fermented after a few days, the flavor is at its prime at about two weeks. It's totally normal to see small bubbles around the surface and even some white foam. Your kraut should not, however, take on a dark color or grow moldy. Keeping the kraut submerged under the brine is the best way to ensure that doesn't happen.

MAKES ABOUT 1 QUART (946 ML)

1 small head green cabbage, about 2 pounds (900 g)

1 tablespoon (15 g) kosher or (18 g) pickling salt

2 teaspoons caraway seeds (optional)

Distilled water, for jarring

1. Remove the soft outer leaves of the cabbage and set aside. Cut the cabbage in quarters, through the stem, and then remove the core from each wedge. Slice each wedge into thin shreds.

2. Add the cabbage to a large mixing bowl, sprinkle the salt over top, and toss together with your hands. Let it sit until the salt begins to draw the liquid from the vegetables, 20 to 30 minutes.

3. Use your hands to massage the salt into the cabbage. After a few minutes, the cabbage will soften and release more liquid. Continue massaging until the leaves are limp, the volume of cabbage is reduced by about half, and there is liquid in the bottom of the bowl, about 5 minutes. Mix in the caraway seeds, if using.

4. Transfer the cabbage and any accumulated liquid to a wide-mouth, quart-size (946 ml) canning jar. Use the back of your hand to firmly press the cabbage down into the jar to release any air and submerge under the liquid. If necessary, add just enough distilled water to completely cover the cabbage, leaving at least 1 inch (2.5 cm) of headspace. Place a reserved outer cabbage leaf over the shredded cabbage to weigh it down and keep it submerged.

5. Tightly seal the jar and leave it in a cool, dark place away from direct sunlight for at least 3 days. Open the jar daily to release any built-up gas from fermentation, taste the kraut, and push the kraut below the surface of the liquid, if necessary. You may see bubbles around the surface, which is a totally normal effect of the fermentation process. Once it has a flavor you enjoy, remove the cabbage leaf at the top of the jar and store the sealed jar in the refrigerator for up to 3 months.

Ginger-Carrot Kraut

There's a vendor at my local farmers market who makes the best selection of krauts and fermented vegetables. This sharp and spicy kraut is inspired by one from their lineup and gets some extra-bold flavor from fresh ginger and garlic. As with all krauts and fermented vegetables, this blend will pick up a tangy flavor starting after a couple days, will get stronger each day it ferments, and is ready for eating as soon as it tastes good to you.

MAKES 1 QUART (946 ML)

½ small head cabbage (about 3 cups [210 g])

3 cups (330 g) packed shredded carrots

1 piece (2 inches, or 5 cm) of fresh ginger, finely chopped

2 cloves garlic, chopped

1 tablespoon (15 g) kosher or (18 g) pickling salt

Distilled water as necessary, for jarring

1. Remove the soft outer leaves of the cabbage and set aside. Cut the cabbage in quarters, through the stem, and then remove the core from each wedge. Slice each wedge into thin shreds.

2. Add the cabbage, carrots, ginger, and garlic to a large bowl. Coat the vegetables well with salt. Let it sit until the salt begins to draw the liquid from the vegetables, 20 to 30 minutes.

3. Massage the salt into the vegetables until the volume is reduced by about half, about 5 minutes.

4. Transfer the vegetables and any accumulated liquid into a wide-mouth quart-size (946 ml) canning jar. Firmly press the vegetables below the surface of the liquid. If necessary, add just enough distilled water to completely cover the vegetables, leaving at least 1 inch (2.5 cm) of headspace. Place a reserved outer cabbage leaf over the vegetables to weigh them down and keep them submerged.

5. Tightly seal the jar and leave it in a cool, dark place away from direct sunlight for at least 3 days. Open the jar daily to release any built-up gas from fermentation, taste the kraut, and push the kraut below the surface of the liquid, if necessary. You may see bubbles around the surface, which is totally normal in the fermentation process. Once the kraut has a flavor you enjoy, remove the cabbage leaf from the top of the jar and store the sealed jar in the refrigerator for up to 3 months.

Lacto-Fermented Mixed Vegetables

Fermenting is not just for cabbage. While firm vegetables like the radishes, carrots, and cauliflower used here are the best choices for fermenting, the process will work with just about any type of vegetable. Consider this recipe your basic template for getting started. As with other ferments, there's no specific time for when the vegetables are ready for eating—it's all a matter of preference and what tastes good to you, although a few days will give you a wonderfully zesty flavor. Do be sure to open the jar once a day to release any built-up gas and give the veggies a taste while you're at it.

MAKES ABOUT 1 QUART (946 ML)

1 quart (946 ml) distilled water

3 tablespoons (45 g) kosher or (54 g) pickling salt

1 small bunch radishes, trimmed and halved

2 medium carrots, peeled and cut into ½-inch (1.3 cm) -thick slices

½ small head cauliflower, cut into small florets

2 cloves garlic, smashed

2 bay leaves

½ teaspoon coriander seeds

½ teaspoon yellow mustard seeds

⅛ teaspoon red pepper flakes (optional)

1. Stir the distilled water and salt together in a large measuring cup or bowl until the salt is dissolved.

2. Add the radishes, carrots, cauliflower, garlic, bay leaves, coriander seeds, mustard seeds, and red pepper flakes, if using, to a wide-mouth 2-quart (1.9 L) canning jar (or divide between two 1-quart [946 ml] jars). Then pour the salt-water solution over top, leaving at least 1 inch (2.5 cm) of headspace. Tightly seal the jar and leave it in a cool, dark place away from direct sunlight for up to 3 days.

3. Open the jar once a day to release any built-up gas from fermentation and taste the vegetables. There is no set time for when the vegetables are done and ready to eat—it is simply a matter of taste. The vegetables will be mild at first and take on a more tangy, funky taste day by day as they continue to ferment.

4. When the vegetables taste good to you, store the sealed jar in the refrigerator for up to 3 months.

Easy Kimchi

When you're ready to move beyond basic krauts, I strongly suggest giving kimchi a try. There are some slight differences in the process, but making kimchi is pretty close to making sauerkraut and other fermented vegetables. It's helpful to wear gloves while mixing the kimchi (a simple pair of thin latex gloves will do), both to prevent the gochugaru from burning your hands and to keep the funky smell from permeating your skin, which can stick around for a while. The amount of time you leave the kimchi to ferment is up to you; it all comes down to how you like the taste. Check and taste the kimchi daily. It's done and ready to be used and eaten as soon as you are happy with the flavor. The longer you ferment, the more intense the kimchi's flavor will be, while the vegetables become softer. Don't be alarmed if you notice small bubbles on the surface of the kimchi—it's a sign the fermentation process is going well.

MAKES ABOUT 1 QUART (946 ML)

1 medium head Napa cabbage (2 to 3 pounds [900 g to 1.4 kg])

¼ cup (60 g) coarse kosher or (72 g) pickling salt

Distilled or filtered water

5 cloves garlic, minced

2 tablespoons (16 g) finely grated ginger

2 tablespoons (18 g) gochugaru (Korean chili powder) or ¼ cup (14 g) red pepper flakes

1 tablespoon (15 ml) Asian fish sauce (optional)

1 teaspoon granulated sugar

2 cups (220 g) shredded carrot (or 1 large carrot, peeled and julienned)

1 bunch scallions, chopped

1. Remove the soft outer leaves of the cabbage. Slice the cabbage lengthwise into quarters and remove the core from each wedge. Chop each wedge into 2-inch (5 cm) pieces and transfer to a large bowl.

2. Sprinkle the cabbage with the salt and use your hands to massage it into the leaves until they begin to wilt. Add just enough cold distilled water to cover the cabbage. The cabbage will float to the surface of the water. Place a large plate over the cabbage to help submerge it under the water. Let it sit for 2 hours.

3. Drain the cabbage, reserving up to 1 cup (235 ml) of the saltwater brine, and then thoroughly rinse the cabbage in a colander under cool water. Set aside.

4. In the same large bowl, mix together the garlic, ginger, gochugaru, fish sauce, if using, and sugar to make a paste.

5. Return the cabbage to the bowl with the chili-paste mixture and add the carrots and scallions. With gloved hands, thoroughly work the chili paste into the vegetables until well coated. Transfer the vegetables to a wide-mouth 2-quart (1.9 L) canning jar (or divide between two 1-quart [946 ml] jars) and use your hands to press down firmly so that the brine covers the vegetables. If necessary, pour just enough of the reserved saltwater brine over the vegetables to cover, leaving 1 inch (2.5 cm) of head space at the top of the jar. Seal tightly and store at room temperature, away from direct sunlight, for 2 to 5 days.

6. Check the kimchi every day to release built-up gas from the jar, push the vegetables below the brine if necessary, and taste the kimchi. It is ready when it tastes good to you.

7. Store the sealed jar in the refrigerator for up to 3 months.

Fermented Salsa

On the surface, this salsa looks just like pico de gallo, the fresh, simple salsa made with tomato, onion, jalapeño, and cilantro. But take a bite, and you'll see there's much more to it. After a few days of lacto-fermentation, this salsa picks up a tangy bite that gets bolder the longer it is fermented. Don't be put off by all the salt—it draws liquid from the ingredients and is necessary for the fermentation process.

MAKES ABOUT 3 CUPS (700 ML)

2 large, ripe tomatoes, cored and diced

1 medium onion, diced

1 jalapeño, seeded and diced

1 clove garlic, minced

½ cup (8 g) packed chopped cilantro leaves

Juice from 1 lime

2 teaspoons kosher salt

1. Mix all the ingredients together in a large bowl, pressing gently to draw out liquid from the vegetables.

2. Transfer to a wide-mouth 1-quart (946 ml) canning jar. Use the back of your hand or a spoon to push the salsa down, to remove any air in the bottom of the jar, and to submerge the vegetables beneath the liquid.

3. Tightly seal the jar. Leave it in a cool, dark place away from direct sunlight for up to 3 days. Check daily and push the salsa below the surface of the liquid, if necessary. When it's ready, the salsa will have small bubbles around the surface and a zesty flavor.

4. Once it has a flavor you enjoy, store the sealed container in the refrigerator for up to 3 months.

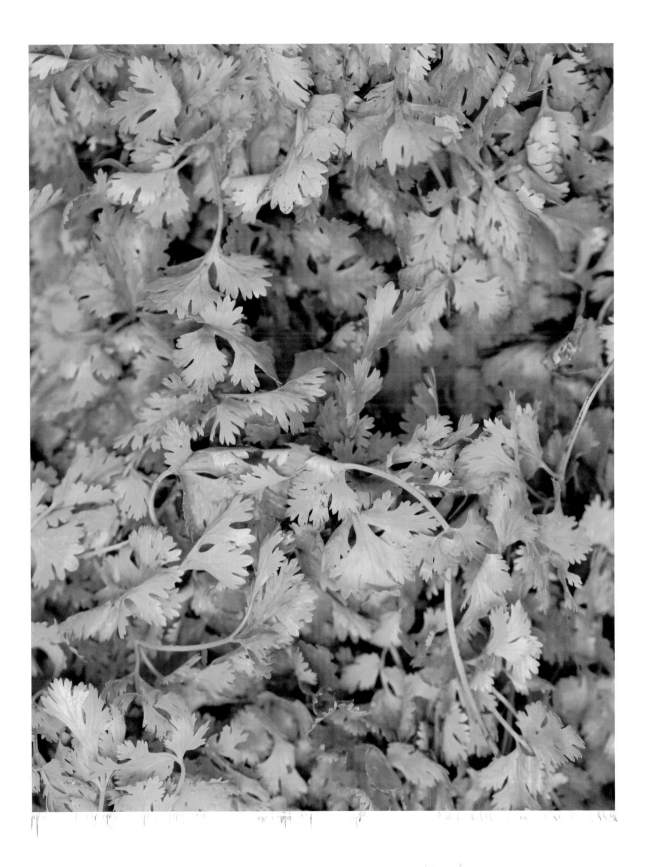

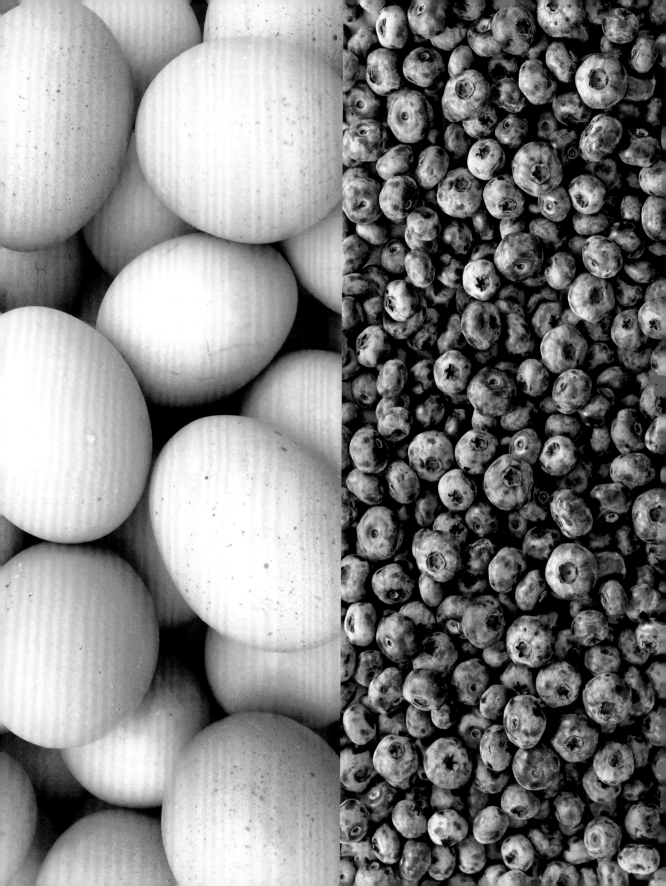

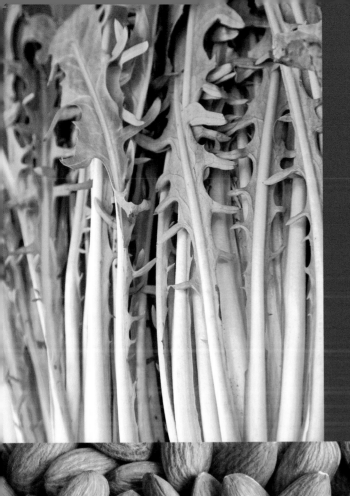

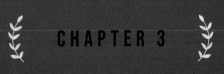
Breakfasts

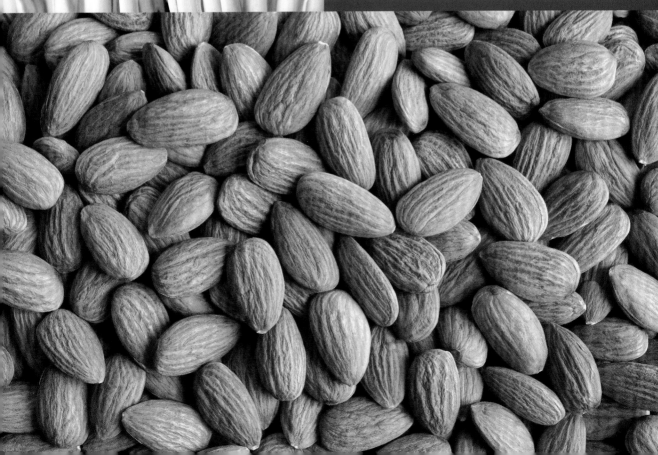

Kefir Bowls *with* Blueberry-Coriander Compote

I'll tell you what makes kefir for breakfast even better—toppings! It's the number-one reason to serve it in a bowl rather than drinking it. And I suggest starting with this simple, spice-kissed fruit compote. I call for blueberries here, which pairs wonderfully with coriander, but you can easily swap in raspberries or blackberries. Just be sure to strain out the seeds. The compote can be made ahead of time and will keep in the refrigerator for up to a week.

SERVES 4

1 cup (145 g) fresh blueberries

1 teaspoon granulated sugar

½ teaspoon ground coriander

2 cups (475 ml) live-culture plain milk kefir, preferably whole milk

SUGGESTED TOPPINGS:
  sliced banana, fresh berries, granola, bee pollen

1. Cook the blueberries and sugar in a small saucepan over medium heat for 5 minutes, stirring regularly with a wooden spoon to mash the berries. The fruit will be broken down and thick. Remove from the heat, stir in the coriander, and cool completely.

2. To serve, divide the kefir among four bowls. Swirl a spoonful of blueberry compote into four bowls. Top with banana, additional berries, granola, and bee pollen, as desired.

Kimchi *and* Avocado Omelet

After partnering kimchi and sliced avocado with my scrambled eggs for quite some time, I had an aha moment and realized that they would also make an unexpectedly delicious omelet filling. You probably haven't considered stuffing funky kimchi inside your omelet but trust me—try it and you won't be disappointed. Added at the very end of cooking, kimchi keeps its slightly crunchy texture, and the tart flavor is just the right contrast to creamy eggs. Kimchi is packed with probiotics, while avocado and scallion give breakfast a boost of prebiotics.

SERVES 1

2 large eggs

1 tablespoon (15 ml) whole or 2% milk

⅛ teaspoon kosher salt

1 scallion, thinly sliced

½ tablespoon unsalted butter

¼ cup (25 g) kimchi, drained and chopped

Sliced avocado, for serving

Toasted sesame seeds, for serving

1. Whisk together the eggs, milk, and salt in a medium bowl until the whites and yolks are completely mixed and the eggs are a bit frothy. Stir in the scallions.

2. Melt the butter in an 8-inch (20 cm) nonstick pan over medium-low heat and swirl the butter around the bottom of the pan so it's fully coated. Pour the eggs into the pan and tilt so the eggs evenly coat the bottom.

3. Gently ease a spatula under the edges of the cooked eggs, lifting and tilting the pan to allow the uncooked eggs to run under the cooked part. Cook until the edges are set and the center is wet but no longer loose or runny, about 2 minutes.

4. Remove the pan from the heat. Spoon the kimchi over one half of the omelet. Use the spatula to gently fold the other half of the omelet over the kimchi. Slide the omelet onto a plate. Top with sliced avocado and sesame seeds.

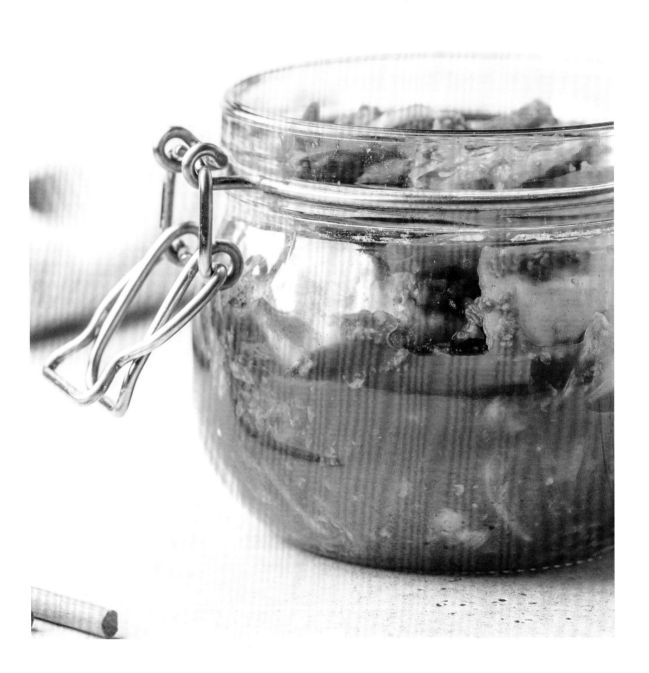

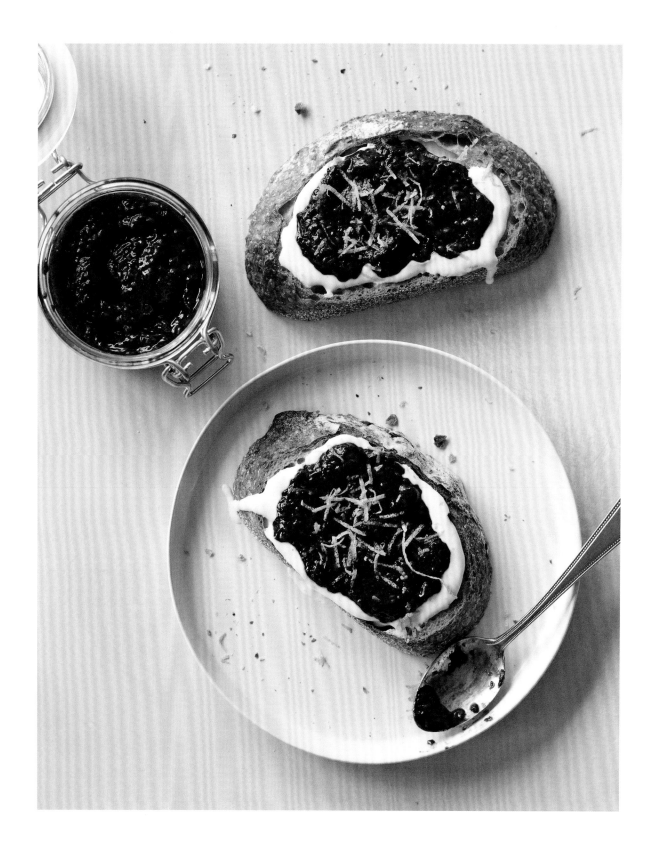

Sourdough *with* Whipped Cottage Cheese *and* Raspberry Chia Jam

If you're a cottage cheese skeptic, I speak from experience when I say that this fancy toast is a terrific introduction. Whirled in the food processor, its once curd-like texture becomes light, fluffy, and wonderfully whipped. And its neutral, creamy flavor is the perfect balance to the tart sweetness of the berries.

SERVES 4

1 cup (140 g) frozen raspberries

1 tablespoon (13 g) chia seeds

2 teaspoons honey, preferably raw

1 teaspoon freshly squeezed lemon juice

Pinch kosher salt

1 cup (255 g) cultured cottage cheese

2 slices thick-cut sourdough or sprouted grain bread, lightly toasted

Finely grated lemon zest, for topping

1. Heat the raspberries in a small saucepan over medium-high heat, stirring occasionally, until bubbling. Break up the fruit with the back of a spoon. Stir in the chia seeds, honey, lemon juice, and salt. Remove from the heat and cool completely, about 10 minutes. The jam will thicken as it cools.

2. Meanwhile, add the cottage cheese to a food processor, regular blender, or use an immersion blender and blend until smooth and creamy, about 2 minutes.

3. Spread the cottage cheese over each piece of toast, top with a layer of raspberry chia jam, and sprinkle with lemon zest.

Cooking Tip!

Mornings can be busy, but I have good news—both the chia jam and whipped cottage cheese can be made ahead of time! Store them separately in covered containers in the refrigerator for up to five days.

Probiotic Breakfast Bowls

You'll find me eating a version of this bowl nearly every day. With a little bit of everything—whole grains, sautéed greens, a yolky egg, creamy yogurt, avocado, and just enough kraut to grace every bite—it's my ideal breakfast. A scoop of kraut (I recommend red cabbage kraut, though you really can't go wrong with any variety) gives this bowl a big pop of flavor to balance the richness of the runny egg yolk and yogurt. Get a head start on breakfast by making the quinoa the night before.

SERVES 4

1 cup (173 g) uncooked quinoa, rinsed

1¾ cups (410 ml) water

Kosher salt

2 tablespoons (28 ml) extra-virgin olive oil, divided

4 cups (120 g) packed baby spinach

4 large eggs

1 cup (240 g) fermented red cabbage kraut

1 avocado, peeled, pitted, and thinly sliced

1 cup (230 g) live-culture plain Greek yogurt, preferably whole milk

2 scallions, thinly sliced

4 teaspoons (12 g) hemp seeds

1. Combine the quinoa, water, and a generous pinch of salt in a medium saucepan. Bring to a boil and then reduce the heat to a simmer and cook, uncovered, until tender, 10 to 12 minutes. Remove from the heat, cover with a lid, and steam for 5 minutes.

2. Heat ½ tablespoon of the oil in a large skillet until shimmering. Add the spinach and cook, tossing frequently, until wilted, 1 to 2 minutes. Divide the spinach among four bowls and wipe the pan clean.

3. Heat the remaining 1½ tablespoons (25 ml) of oil in the skillet over medium heat. Crack the eggs into the skillet and season each one with a pinch of salt. Cook until the edges are crisp and the whites are set, about 3 minutes.

4. Divide the quinoa among the bowls. Top with each with a fried egg, kraut, avocado slices, a scoop of yogurt, scallions, and hemp seeds.

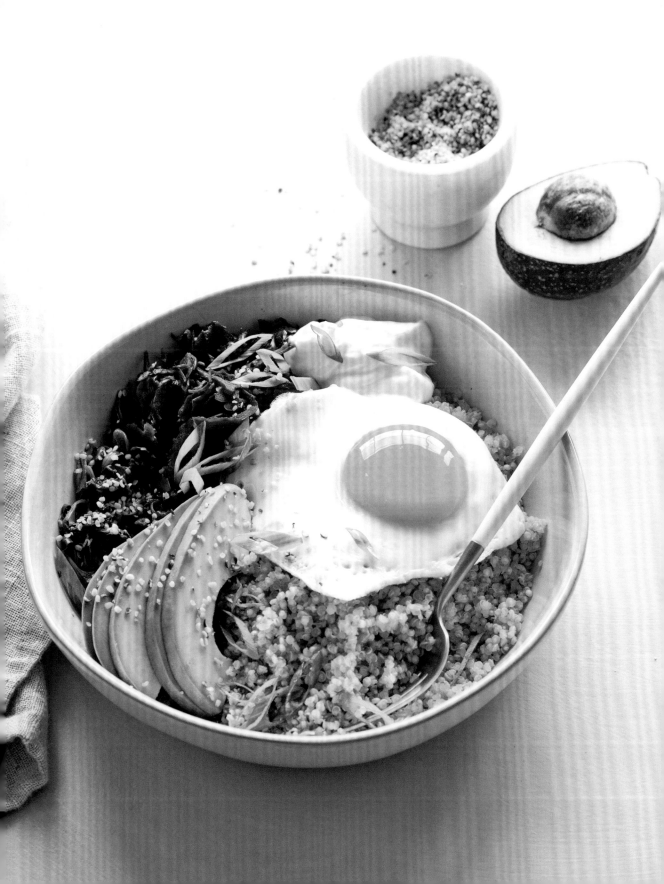

Breakfast Burritos *with* Scrambled Tofu *and* Fermented Salsa

Crumbled tofu replaces eggs in this protein-packed, handheld breakfast. It takes on a texture akin to scrambled eggs, with a hint of warm spice and cheesiness from nutritional yeast. It's worth making a batch of fermented salsa (page 38) at home (which keeps for months in the refrigerator), though you can also check your local health food store or fermented foods seller for a premade version. In addition to the probiotic-rich fermented salsa and yogurt, avocado and raw scallions also bring some prebiotics to breakfast.

SERVES 4

14 ounces (390 g) extra-firm tofu, pressed and drained

1 tablespoon (15 ml) extra-virgin olive oil

2 tablespoons (8 g) nutritional yeast

1 teaspoon chili powder

1 teaspoon ground cumin

1 teaspoon kosher salt

¼ teaspoon freshly ground black pepper

1 cup (240 g) black beans, drained and rinsed

2 cups (60 g) baby spinach

½ cup (115 ml) live-culture plain Greek yogurt, preferably whole milk

4 large flour tortillas

2 scallions, thinly sliced

1 avocado, peeled, pitted, and thinly sliced

½ cup (120 ml) fermented salsa (page 38)

1. Add the tofu to a medium bowl and break into small curds with a fork or your fingers. Heat the oil in a large skillet over medium-high heat. Add the tofu and sauté for 2 minutes.

2. Stir in the nutritional yeast, chili powder, cumin, salt, and pepper until well combined and continue cooking until the tofu is lightly browned, 4 to 5 minutes. Stir in the black beans and spinach and cook until the beans are heated through and the spinach is wilted, about 2 minutes more.

3. Spread the yogurt over the tortillas and then top with scrambled tofu, scallions, sliced avocado, and salsa. Fold the sides and bottom of the tortilla over the filling and roll it up.

Orange-Tahini Overnight Oats

If you believe peanut or almond butter is a must with oatmeal, nutty tahini is a fun way to change up your breakfast routine. It's mixed in with the oats, but it's also worth an extra drizzle over the top of the bowl when you're dishing it out. The oats will last for a couple days and are on the thick side, but they can be easily thinned out with a splash of milk when serving.

SERVES 4 TO 6

2 cups (192 g) whole rolled oats

2 tablespoons (14 g) ground flaxseed

2 cups (475 ml) milk of choice

1 cup (230 g) live-culture plain Greek yogurt, perferably whole milk

2 tablespoons (40 g) honey, preferably raw

2 tablespoons (30 g) tahini

1 teaspoon ground cinnamon

1 teaspoon vanilla extract

⅛ teaspoon kosher salt

SUGGESTED TOPPINGS:

milk of choice, semented navel orange, pomegranate arils, chopped toasted almonds, tahini

1. Add the oats, flaxseed, milk, yogurt, honey, tahini, cinnamon, vanilla, and salt to a large bowl. Mix until well combined. Cover and refrigerate overnight.

2. To serve, stir the chilled oat mixture once more. Divide it among four to six bowls and top with an extra splash of milk, if desired, along with orange segments, pomegranate arils, almonds, and a drizzle
of tahini.

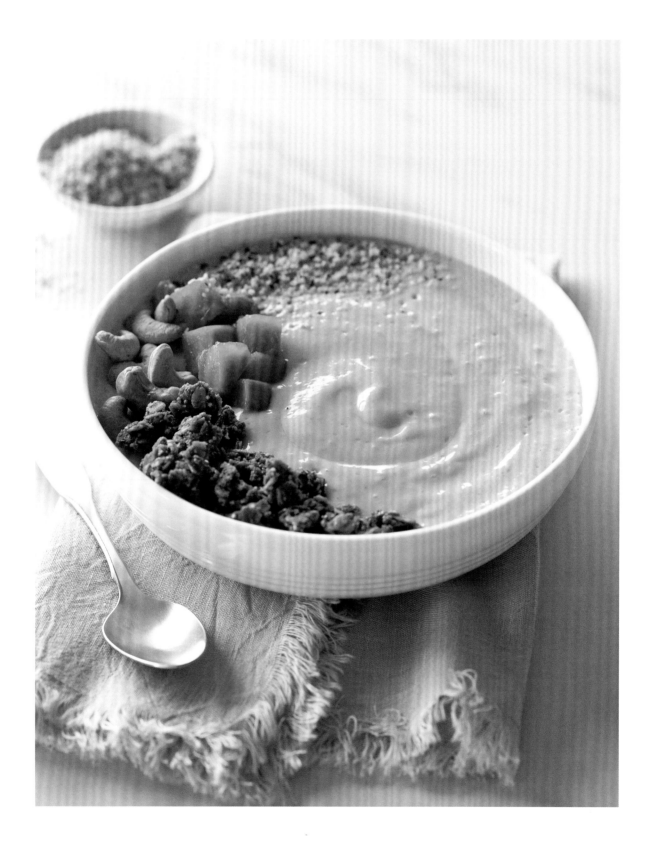

Papaya Lassi Bowls

If you're into yogurt and fruit or smoothies for breakfast, this is such a fun way to change things up. Traditional lassis are an Indian yogurt drink, and this version is blended extra thick with a subtle sweetness and tang from the yogurt, plus a hint of warm spice. It's worth planning ahead and popping the bowls in the freezer the night before—you'll love the extra chill it brings to breakfast.

SERVES 2

3 cups (420 g) cubed papaya (from 1 medium papaya)

1½ cups (345 g) live-culture plain Greek yogurt, preferably whole milk

½ cup (120 ml) whole or 2% milk

2 tablespoons (40 g) honey, preferably raw

½ teaspoon ground cardamom

Pinch kosher salt

SUGGESTED TOPPINGS:
fresh papaya, granola, toasted cashews, hemp seeds

1. Place two individual serving bowls in the freezer while you prepare the lassi. (You can even freeze them the night before.)

2. Add the papaya, yogurt, milk, honey, cardamom, and salt to a blender and process continuously until smooth and creamy. Divide the lassi between the chilled bowls and top with fresh papaya, granola, cashews, and hemp seeds, as desired.

Cultured Cottage Cheese *and* Granola Breakfast Bowls

There are so many ways to work cultured cottage cheese into breakfast, but there is none quite as easy and satisfying as using it just as you would yogurt for a breakfast bowl, loaded with your granola of choice and fresh fruit.

SERVES 2

1½ cups (340 g) cultured cottage
   cheese

½ cup (54 g) granola

Fresh strawberries, sliced

Fresh raspberries

Fresh blueberries

Bee pollen

Fresh mint leaves

1. Divide the cottage cheese between two bowls.

2. Add the granola and any combination of the fresh strawberries, raspberries, and blueberries to the cottage cheese. Top with bee pollen and fresh mint leaves, to taste.

Bircher Muesli *with* Kefir

Since Bircher muesli was first created about 1900, a stream of variations has emerged, and this one is my favorite. It's like overnight oats, but this hearty breakfast dish is just as much about the oats as it is the fruit and nut mix-ins. Kefir adds probiotics and leaves the muesli with a thicker texture than you'd get from milk alone. For an extra boost, pour a splash of kefir over top when serving.

SERVES 4 TO 6

2 cups (192 g) whole rolled oats

1 Granny Smith apple, cored and finely chopped

¼ cup (25 g) chopped toasted almonds

¼ cup (35 g) golden raisins

4 pitted Medjool dates, chopped

½ teaspoon ground cinnamon

Pinch kosher salt

1½ cups (355 ml) live-culture plain milk kefir, preferably whole milk, plus more for serving

1½ cups (355 ml) whole or 2% milk

SUGGESTED TOPPINGS:
unsweetened toasted coconut flakes, toasted pumpkin seeds, honey (preferably raw)

1. Stir together the oats, apple, almonds, raisins, dates, cinnamon, and salt in a large bowl. Pour in the kefir and milk and stir well to combine. Cover and refrigerate overnight.

2. Stir the chilled muesli once more before serving and then divide among four to six bowls. Add extra kefir and coconut flakes, pumpkin seeds, or honey, as desired, and serve.

Scrambled Eggs *and* Dandelion Greens *with* Herbed Cheese *on* Toast

This fast but satisfying breakfast combines my two preferred ways to eat toast: partnered with scrambled eggs and slathered with a simple, delicious spread to make it feel more elegant. Cultured soft farmer cheese has a texture that might remind you of ricotta and a mild flavor that makes it the perfect blank slate for a mess of fresh herbs and garlic. Everything gets piled on a slice of crusty sourdough, and it's up to you whether you eat it with your hands or grab a fork and knife.

SERVES 4

6 ounces (170 g) cultured farmer cheese (see page 20)

2 tablespoons (8 g) finely chopped fresh parsley

2 tablespoons (6 g) snipped chives

1 clove garlic, minced

¾ teaspoon kosher salt, divided

8 large eggs

2 tablespoons (28 ml) extra-virgin olive oil

4 cups (220 g) packed chopped dandelion greens (1 small bunch)

4 slices sourdough or sprouted grain bread, lightly toasted

1. Add the farmer cheese, parsley, chives, garlic, and ¼ teaspoon of the salt to a medium bowl and mash together with a fork to combine. Set aside.

2. Add the eggs to a large bowl and whisk until the yolks and whites are well combined and frothy. Whisk in the remaining ½ teaspoon of salt.

3. Heat the oil in a large skillet over medium-low heat until shimmering. Add the greens and cook, tossing occasionally, until wilted, about 5 minutes.

4. Reduce the heat to low and pour in the eggs. Cook, undisturbed, until the eggs begin to set around the edge of the pan. Use a rubber spatula to gently push the eggs around, scraping the cooked eggs from the bottom of the pan, until they're cooked through but not dry. Remove the pan from the heat.

5. Spread a thin, even layer of the herbed cheese over the toasted sourdough and then divide the eggs and greens among each slice of bread.

Breakfast Salad *with* Kombucha Vinaigrette

If you feel a little skeptical about salad for breakfast, I get it. There was a time when I was in your shoes, too. But believe me—give it a chance and this version, with its runny egg, ripe blueberries, creamy avocado, bitter greens, and zesty probiotic vinaigrette, will make you a believer. Save some time in the morning by cooking the quinoa and whisking together the dressing the night before.

SERVES 4

4 large eggs

4 ounces (115 g) dandelion greens, chopped

4 ounces (115 g) arugula

½ cup (93 g) cooked quinoa

½ cup (75 g) blueberries

½ cup (58 g) thinly sliced red onion

1 avocado, peeled, pitted, and chopped

½ cup (120 ml) Kombucha Vinaigrette (page 91), divided

¼ cup (30 g) chopped toasted walnuts

1. Bring a medium saucepan of water to a low boil over medium-high heat. Gently add the eggs and cook for 6 or 7 minutes. Use a slotted spoon to transfer the eggs to an ice bath to stop the cooking and chill for 5 minutes. The eggs will still be slightly warm. Carefully peel the eggs and slice them in half.

2. Meanwhile, add the dandelion greens, arugula, quinoa, blueberries, onion, and avocado to a large bowl. Drizzle with ¼ cup (60 ml) of the Kombucha Vinaigrette and toss to combine. Divide among four plates or shallow bowls and then top with an egg, walnuts, and additional Kombucha Vinaigrette.

Blueberries and Cream Overnight Oats

The second those overflowing baskets of blueberries hit the farmers market every spring, this breakfast is always at the top of my list. Mixed together in advance and soaked overnight, the combo of milk and yogurt softens the oats, leaving you with a creamy, subtly sweet breakfast. I prefer Greek yogurt for the extra-rich consistency and the protein boost but know that regular unsweetened yogurt works just as well here. Oats and flaxseed are also a great source of prebiotic fiber.

SERVES 4 TO 6

2 cups (192 g) whole rolled oats

1 cup (145 g) fresh or frozen blueberries

2 tablespoons (26 g) chia seeds

2 tablespoons (14 g) ground flaxseed

2½ cups (570 ml) milk of choice

1 cup (230 g) live-culture plain Greek yogurt, preferably whole milk

2 tablespoons (28 ml) pure maple syrup or (40 g) honey, preferably raw

1 teaspoon vanilla extract

⅛ teaspoon kosher salt

SUGGESTED TOPPINGS

live-culture plain Greek yogurt, fresh or frozen blueberries, sliced banana, toasted pecans

1. Combine the oats, blueberries, chia seeds, flaxseed, milk, yogurt, maple syrup or honey, vanilla, and salt in a large bowl and mix until well combined. Cover the oat mixture and refrigerate overnight.

2. To serve, stir the chilled oats once more. Divide it among four to six bowls and top with a dollop of yogurt, some blueberries, sliced banana, and a few pecans, if desired.

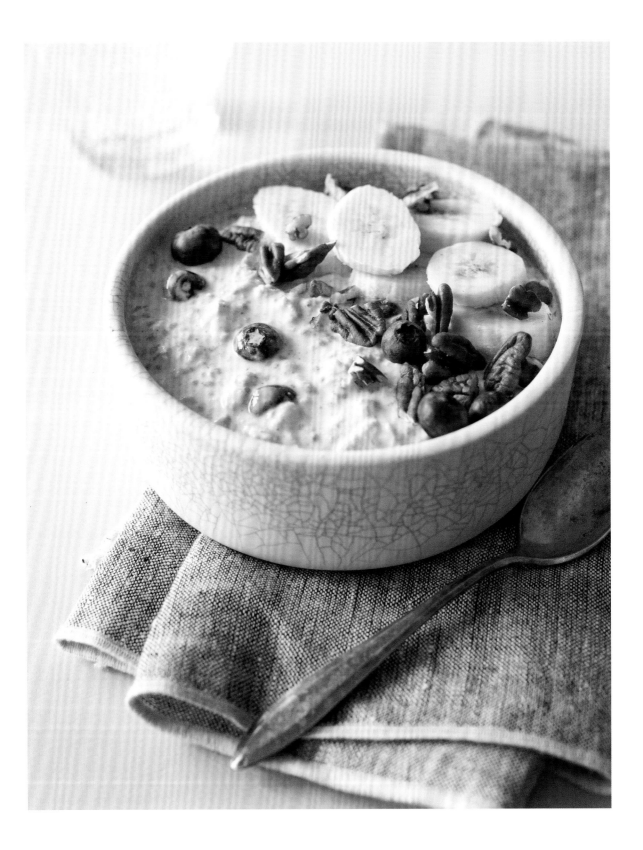

Creamy Breakfast Barley

If you love waking up to a bowl of warm, creamy oatmeal, it's time to give barley a try at breakfast time. Not only does it pack in even more protein, but it's a great source of prebiotic fiber. And when it comes to mix-ins, treat this nutty, toothsome breakfast bowl just as you would oats. Everything from a splash of milk to a drizzle of honey or maple syrup and a dollop of probiotic-rich yogurt or kefir are all fair game.

SERVES 4

2¼ cups (535 ml) water

¾ cup (150 g) pearl barley

¼ teaspoon kosher salt

1 cup (235 ml) milk of choice

1 teaspoon garam masala

1 cup (170 g) probiotic coconut yogurt

½ cup (65 g) chopped dried apricots

¼ cup (31 g) toasted chopped pistachios

2 tablespoons (40 g) honey, preferably raw

1. Combine the water, barley, and salt in a medium saucepan. Bring to a boil and then reduce the heat, cover, and simmer until tender and the water has been absorbed, about 30 minutes. Stir in the milk and garam masala and simmer for another 2 minutes.

2. Divide the barley among four bowls. Top with a dollop of coconut yogurt, dried apricots, pistachios, and a drizzle of honey.

Ingredient Tip: Hulled vs. Pearl Barley

You'll notice that all the barley recipes in the book called for pearl barley, which is not the same as hulled barley. Pearl barley is the most common type of barley and the quicker cooking of the two, as the outer hull and bran layers of the grain have been removed. Hulled barley, in contrast, is minimally processed with only the inedible, outer hull removed, and takes considerably longer to cook.

Turkish-Style Fried Eggs *with* Yogurt

For this dish, I like to pop the pitas in a warm oven on very low heat while I prepare the yogurt spread and cook the eggs. By the time I'm ready to assemble breakfast, the pitas are warmed through and pillowy soft with lightly crisped edges. If you're not already familiar with it, Aleppo pepper is a super-flavorful Middle Eastern spice with earthy undertones and a gentle heat that's a touch gentler than red pepper flakes.

SERVES 4

1 cup (230 g) live-culture plain
   Greek yogurt, preferably
   whole milk

2 tablespoons (8 g) finely chopped
   fresh dill

1 tablespoon (15 ml) freshly
   squeezed lemon juice

1 clove garlic, minced

½ teaspoon kosher salt, plus more
   for the eggs

2 tablespoons (28 ml) extra-virgin
   olive oil, plus more as needed

8 large eggs

4 whole wheat pitas, warmed

1 teaspoon Aleppo pepper

1. Stir together the yogurt, dill, lemon juice, garlic, and salt in a medium bowl. Set aside.

2. Heat the oil in a large nonstick skillet over medium-high heat until shimmering. Working in batches and adding more oil if necessary, gently crack the eggs into the skillet and sprinkle with salt. Cook until the egg whites are set, the edges are lacey, and the yolks are still runny.

3. Divide the pita bread among four plates and spread a layer of the herbed yogurt over each. Carefully top each pita with two eggs and sprinkle with the Aleppo pepper.

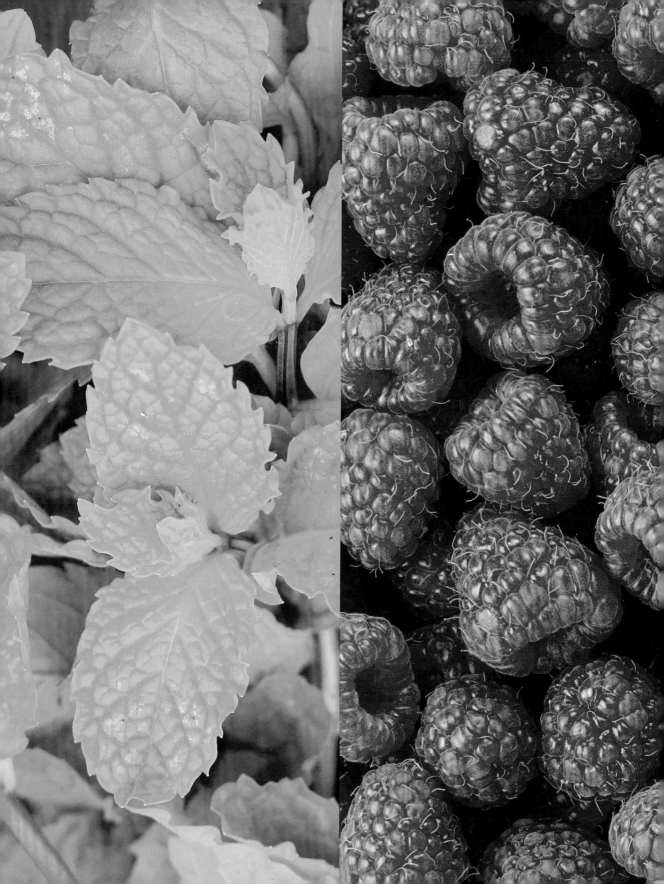

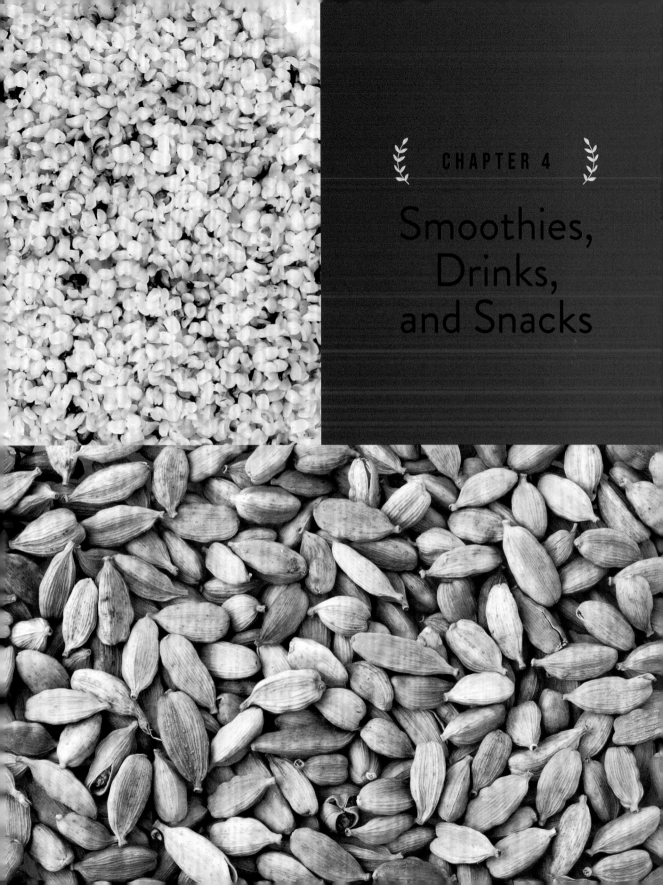

CHAPTER 4

Smoothies,
Drinks,
and Snacks

Mango-Ginger Smoothie

When I was pregnant with my son, this just-sweet-enough smoothie almost single-handedly got me through the first trimester, when there were very few things I was able to stomach for breakfast. I could be sure the ginger would calm my stomach and felt good about getting a regular boost of protein and probiotics from Greek yogurt. If you enjoy the kick of fresh ginger, don't be afraid to add a little more (or tone it down if you prefer a milder flavor).

SERVES 2

2 cups (475 ml) coconut water

¾ cup (180 g) live-culture plain Greek yogurt, preferably whole milk

2 medium frozen bananas, chopped

1½ cups (281 g) frozen mango chunks

1 tablespoon (7 g) ground flaxseed

1 piece (2 inches or 5 cm) fresh ginger, peeled and chopped

Pinch kosher salt

1. Add all the ingredients to a blender and blend on high speed until the consistency is smooth and creamy.

2. Divide the smoothie between two tall, preferably chilled glasses and serve immediately.

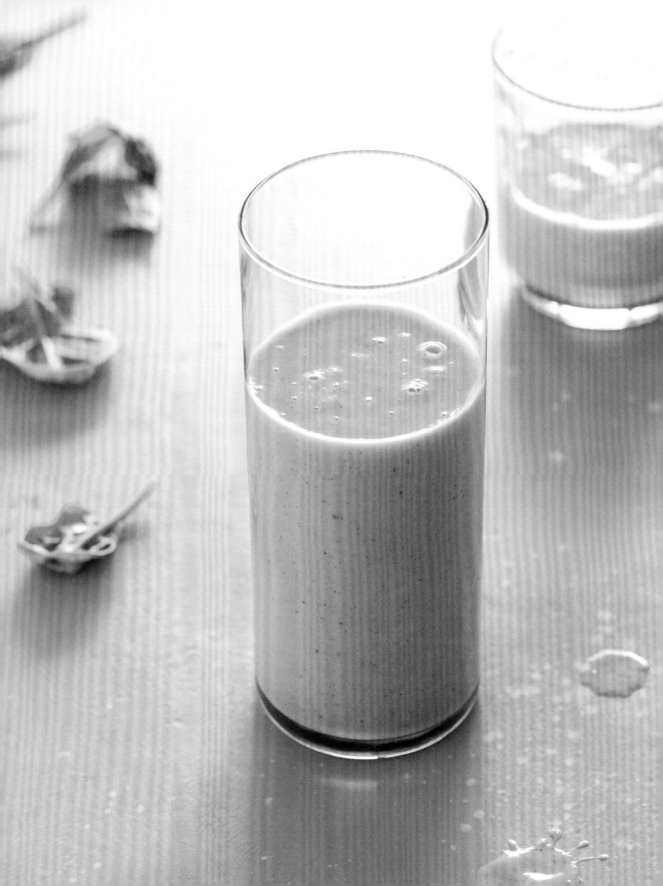

Tropical Green Smoothie

While this creamy smoothie is a regular in my breakfast rotation throughout the year, I appreciate it especially on cold, dreary winter mornings. Greek yogurt lends a boost of protein and probiotics and when combined with prebiotic-friendly avocado, also makes for an extra-smooth and creamy texture. If you don't have frozen mango handy, go ahead and double down on the pineapple.

SERVES 2

2 cups (475 ml) coconut water

1 cup (230 g) live-culture plain Greek yogurt, preferably whole milk

1½ cups (45 g) packed baby spinach

1 cup (187 g) frozen pineapple chunks

1 cup (187 g) frozen mango chunks

1 medium frozen banana, chopped

½ ripe avocado, peeled and pitted

1 pitted Medjool date

¼ cup (9 g) fresh mint leaves

Pinch kosher salt

1. Add all the ingredients to a blender and blend on high speed until the consistency is smooth and creamy.

2. Divide the smoothie between two tall, preferably chilled glasses and serve immediately.

Mixed-Berry Probiotic Power Smoothie

There are smoothies that make a good snack and those that are undeniably meal worthy. This one falls firmly into the latter category. With creamy kefir as the base, not only does it offer you get a big dose of probiotics, but it also has a hint of sweetness with lots of body. It contains ingredients unexpected in a smoothie, such as cauliflower and baby spinach, that give it an interesting depth. Plus, along with the nut butter and hemp seeds, it packs plenty of protein to keep you satisfied.

SERVES 2

2 cups (475 ml) live-culture plain milk kefir, preferably whole milk

2 cups (280 g) frozen mixed berries

1 cup (132 g) frozen small cauliflower florets

1 cup (30 g) baby spinach

2 tablespoons (32 g) almond butter

2 tablespoons (40 g) honey, preferably raw

2 tablespoons (18 g) hemp seeds

½ teaspoon ground cinnamon

Pinch kosher salt

1. Add all the ingredients to a blender and blend on high speed until the consistency is smooth and creamy.

2. Divide the smoothie between two tall, preferably chilled glasses and serve immediately.

Orange-Pineapple Smoothie

Remember that age-old saying about not judging a book by its cover? Well, that goes for this smoothie. It blends up with a milky, creamy appearance, yet surprises your tongue with a bright, fun flavor. It's a hit especially during those drab winter months when you crave a dose of sunshine. The Greek yogurt and chia seeds add a punch of protein, while the banana adds a nice dose of prebiotics.

SERVES 2

1½ cups (355 ml) orange juice

¾ cup (180 g) live-culture plain Greek yogurt, preferably whole milk

1½ cups (281 g) frozen pineapple chunks

1 medium frozen banana, chopped

2 tablespoons (26 g) chia seeds

Pinch kosher salt

1. Add all the ingredients to a blender and blend on high speed until the consistency is smooth and creamy.

2. Divide the smoothie between two tall, preferably chilled glasses and serve immediately.

Beet-Raspberry Smoothie

There's no question that vibrant yet earthy beets can be a bit polarizing. But partnering them with sweet berries and dates, plus adding the richness of milky kefir, really mellows their flavor, keeping them from overpowering this stunning smoothie.

SERVES 2

1 cup (235 ml) unsweetened almond or cashew milk

1 cup (235 ml) live-culture plain milk kefir, preferably whole milk

2 pitted Medjool dates

2 cups (280 g) frozen raspberries

1 small beet, peeled and shredded (about ½ cup [113 g])

1 tablespoon (7 g) ground flaxseed

1 tablespoon (13 g) chia seeds

Pinch kosher salt

1. Add all the ingredients to a blender and blend on high speed until the consistency is smooth and creamy.

2. Divide the smoothie between two tall, preferably chilled glasses and serve immediately.

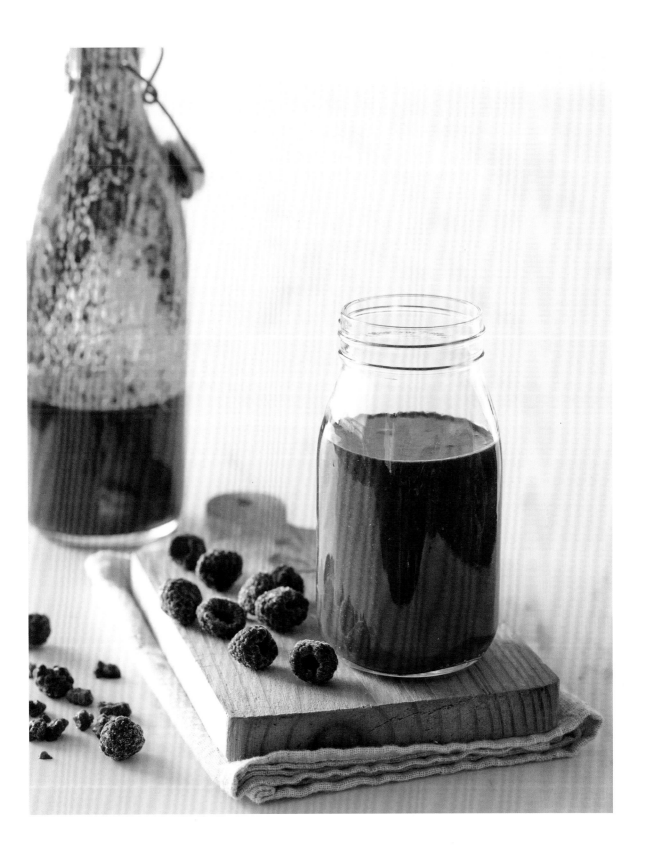

Blueberry-Banana Protein Smoothie

If you're still a little unsure about cottage cheese (and, of course, if you're already a fan), creamy smoothies are a great and easy way to start eating more of it. Not only does cultured cottage cheese work probiotics into breakfast, but it's packed with protein, so you can be certain this smoothie will fill you up. Remember to look for cottage cheese that contains live and active cultures to get the maximum probiotic benefit.

SERVES 2

2 cups (475 ml) unsweetened almond or cashew milk

¾ cup (165 g) cultured cottage cheese

1½ cups (233 g) frozen blueberries

2 medium frozen bananas, chopped

1 tablespoon (20 g) honey, preferably raw

1 tablespoon (13 g) chia seeds

1 tablespoon (7 g) ground flaxseed

½ teaspoon ground cinnamon

Pinch kosher salt

1. Add all the ingredients to a blender and blend on high speed until the consistency is smooth and creamy.

2. Divide the smoothie between two tall, preferably chilled glasses and serve immediately.

Strawberry Almond Protein Smoothie

If you want to take advantage of cottage cheese's health benefits but are unaccustomed to the texture, smoothies are the perfect solution. I should know, I speak from experience. In addition to the probiotics found in cultured cottage cheese, it gives this berry smoothie a shot of protein and an extra-creamy texture.

SERVES 2

2 cups (475 ml) unsweetened almond milk

¾ cup (165 g) cultured cottage cheese

2 tablespoons (32 g) creamy almond butter

2 cups (298 g) frozen strawberries

2 pitted Medjool dates

2 tablespoons (18 g) hemp seeds

1 tablespoon (7 g) ground flaxseed

Pinch kosher salt

1. Add all the ingredients to a blender and blend on high speed until the consistency is smooth and creamy.

2. Divide the smoothie between two tall, preferably chilled glasses and serve immediately.

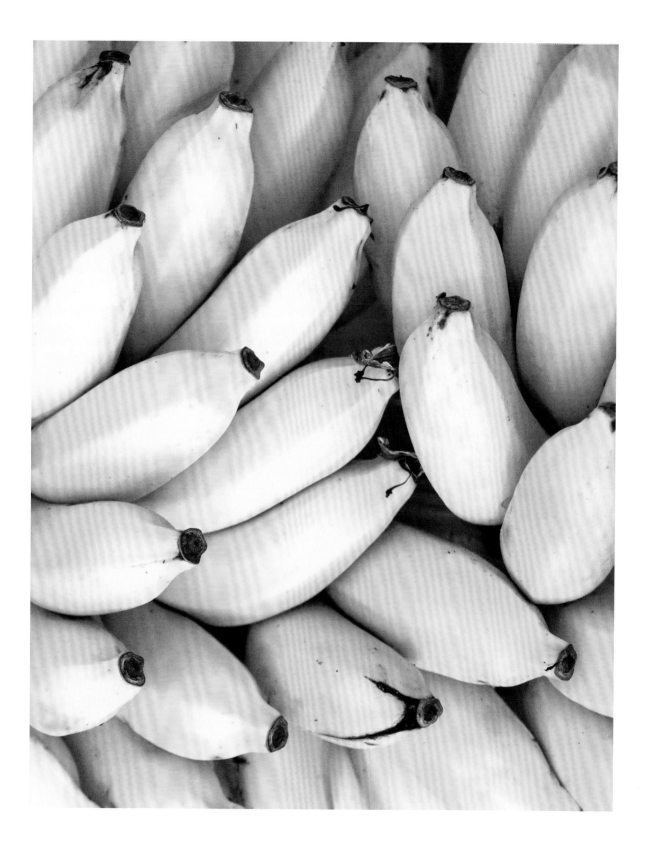

Banana-Cardamom Lassi

As a lassi should be, this subtly sweet drink with warm spiced undertones from the cardamom is nothing short of refreshing. In addition to adding plenty of natural sweetness to the lassi, raw banana is a good source of prebiotics.

SERVES 2

1 large (or 2 small) ripe banana, chopped

1 cup (230 g) live-culture plain Greek yogurt, preferably whole milk

½ cup (120 ml) whole or 2% milk

1 tablespoon (20 g) honey, preferably raw

½ teaspoon ground cardamom

Pinch kosher salt

1. Add all the ingredients to a blender and process continuously until the consistency is smooth and creamy.

2. Divide the smoothie between two chilled glasses. You can also serve over ice, if desired.

Coconut Bliss Smoothie

Calling all coconut lovers—this probiotic-rich smoothie has your name all over it! If you're not yet acquainted, probiotic coconut yogurt has an ultrarich and creamy texture (even more so than Greek yogurt) with a full-on coconut flavor that does not hold back. A squeeze of citrusy lime keeps the richness in check.

SERVES 2

2 cups (475 ml) coconut water

¾ cup (128 g) probiotic coconut
   yogurt

2 medium frozen bananas, chopped

1 cup (132 g) frozen small
   cauliflower florets

2 pitted Medjool dates

Juice of ½ lime

2 tablespoons (32 g) almond butter

1 tablespoon (9 g) hemp seeds

Pinch kosher salt

1. Add all the ingredients to a blender and blend on high speed until the consistency is smooth and creamy.

2. Divide the smoothie between two tall, preferably chilled glasses and serve immediately.

Blood Orange Kefir Lassi

Come the middle of winter, this pretty pale-pink drink is one of the best reasons to keep an eye out for blood oranges, named for their shocking deep red-orange hue. Because this lassi skips the traditional yogurt in favor of milk kefir, you'll notice that it has a thinner consistency. Rest assured, though; it's no less delicious and refreshing. The window for blood oranges can be short, so if you can't get your hands on them, use Cara Cara, satsuma, or navel oranges instead.

SERVES 2

2 blood oranges, peeled, segmented, and pitted

1½ cups (355 ml) live-culture plain milk kefir, preferably whole milk

½ cup (120 ml) ice

2 tablespoons (40 g) honey, preferably raw

½ teaspoon orange blossom water

Pinch kosher salt

1. Add all the ingredients to a blender and process continuously until the consistency is smooth and creamy.

2. Divide the smoothie between two chilled glasses. You can also serve over ice, if desired.

Raspberry-Rose Lassi

A splash of delicate and floral rosewater is what makes this probiotic yogurt drink shine. It's not a traditional addition to a lassi (nor are the raspberries), but it's absolutely delicious nonetheless. Look for rosewater near the spices or in the Middle Eastern section of your grocer.

SERVES 2

1 cup (125 g) fresh raspberries

1 cup (230 ml) live-culture plain Greek yogurt, preferably whole milk

½ cup (235 g) whole or 2% milk

1 tablespoon (20 g) honey, preferably raw

1 teaspoon rosewater

Pinch kosher salt

1. Add all the ingredients to a blender and process continuously until the consistency is smooth and creamy.

2. Divide the smoothie between two chilled glasses. You can also serve over ice, if desired.

Raspberry-Ginger Kombucha Fizz

Let your next bottle of fermented tea serve as the base for a fast yet sophisticated mocktail and you will not be disappointed. It's super fizzy, with just the right amount of natural sweetness from the berries and spice from the ginger beer, while the kombucha gives it a bright twist. The recipe calls for ginger kombucha, though you can easily substitute unflavored kombucha, lemon, or even raspberry. You'll still get the welcome sharp bite of ginger from the ginger beer.

SERVES 4

1 cup (125 g) fresh raspberries, plus more for garnish

½ cup (18 g) fresh mint leaves, plus more for garnish

Crushed ice

16 ounces (475 ml) ginger kombucha

16 ounces (475 ml) ginger beer

1. Divide the raspberries and mint among four glasses and then use a muddler or the back of a spoon to press and combine the fruit and herbs.

2. Top the raspberry-mint mixture with crushed ice, kombucha, and ginger beer and stir to combine. Serve with a sprig of mint and a couple of raspberries as garnish.

Miso-Banana Toast

After years of using a few slices of banana to accompany nut butter as a toast topping, I decided it was high time to make banana shine as the main attraction. Not only is it a nutritious snack, it's also a great source of prebiotics. Banana is paired with probiotic-rich miso paste to give this naturally sweet toast topper a savory twist with a bite of umami.

SERVES 1

1 small (or ½ large) ripe banana, chopped

1 teaspoon white or yellow miso paste

1 slice multigrain toast

SUGGESTED TOPPINGS:
toasted pepitas, cacao nibs, hemp seeds, buckwheat crunch

1. Add the banana and miso paste to a small bowl. Mash with a fork until it is smooth and creamy and the miso is well combined.

2. Evenly spread the banana mixture over the toast. Sprinkle with pepitas, cacao, hemp seeds, or buckwheat, as desired, and serve.

Rice Cake *with* Mashed Avocado *and* Kraut

If there's one thing I love more than avocado toast, it's rice cakes with mashed avocado. The lightness of the rice cakes makes this my perfect afternoon snack, with the fattiness of the avocado just enough to make me feel satisfied. And to keep things interesting, I love topping it with a generous forkful of kraut. Its distinctive flavor makes it the star of this otherwise mild-mannered (prebiotic- and probiotic-rich) snack.

SERVES 2

1 medium ripe avocado, peeled and pitted

2 rice cakes

½ cup (120 g) fermented red cabbage kraut

1 tablespoon (9 g) hemp seeds

1. On a plate or in a small bowl, mash the avocado flesh with a fork or spoon and then spread it evenly over the rice cakes.

2. Top each rice cake with kraut, sprinkle with hemp seeds, and serve.

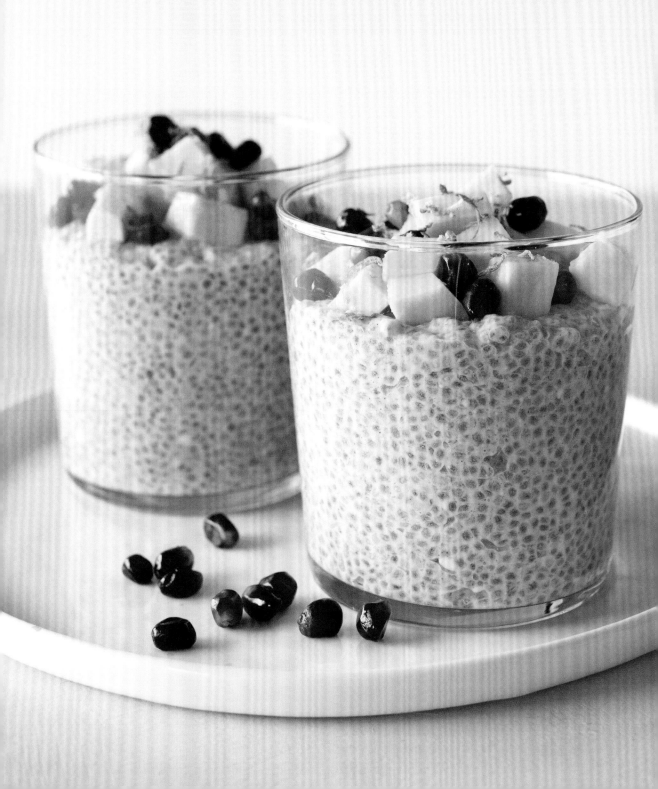

Coconut-Vanilla Chia Pudding

Swapping some of the milk for a generous dollop of probiotic coconut yogurt is my trick for giving creamy chia pudding extra nutritional benefit with probiotics. Unlike traditional coconut yogurt, the probiotic stuff has an ultrathick, luxurious texture with a rich coconut-forward flavor and excellent gut-health benefits.

SERVES 4 TO 6

1 cup (235 ml) unsweetened canned coconut milk

½ cup (120 ml) unsweetened almond milk

½ cup (85 g) probiotic coconut yogurt

2 tablespoons (40 g) honey, preferably raw, or (28 ml) pure maple syrup

2 teaspoons vanilla extract

½ teaspoon ground cinnamon

¼ teaspoon kosher salt

½ cup (104 g) chia seeds

SUGGESTED TOPPINGS:
diced mango, pomegranate arils, lime zest

1. Add the coconut milk, almond milk, yogurt, honey or maple syrup, vanilla, cinnamon, and salt to a large bowl and stir well until smooth.

2. Add the chia seeds and stir well to combine. Cover and refrigerate the pudding overnight.

3. To serve, stir the chilled pudding once more and then divide among four to six bowls. Top with diced mango, pomegranate arils, and lime zest, as desired.

Tangy Deviled Eggs

I think the best way to top off deviled eggs isn't with spices or fresh herbs but with a bite of sauerkraut. I love using red cabbage kraut for the bold pop of color it adds to the eggs, but any variety (along with kimchi) will work well. If your jar of kraut includes extra brine, I highly recommend pouring off a spoonful to mix into the egg yolk filling for a little extra tang.

MAKES 12 EGGS

6 large hard-boiled eggs

⅓ cup (77 g) live-culture plain Greek yogurt, preferably whole milk

1 teaspoon fermented kraut brine (optional)

1 teaspoon Dijon mustard

½ teaspoon kosher salt

¼ teaspoon freshly ground black pepper

¼ cup (60 g) fermented red cabbage kraut

1. Slice the hard-boiled eggs in half lengthwise. Gently scoop out the yolks and add them to a medium bowl. Use a fork to break up the yolks into small crumbles.

2. Add the yogurt, brine (if using), mustard, salt, and pepper to the bowl and mix until well combined and smooth. Transfer the filling to a piping bag.

3. Place the egg whites cut-side up on a large plate or platter. Pipe the filling into the egg whites. Top with kraut just before serving.

Cooking Tip!

I've tried just about every trick out there for cooking and peeling hard-boiled eggs, and this is the simple, foolproof method that works like a charm every single time. Cover the eggs with water in a saucepan, bring to a low boil over medium-low heat, and cook for 6 or 7 minutes. As soon as the time is up, immediately transfer the eggs to an ice bath and let them sit for 5 minutes before peeling. Tap the shells lightly with the dull side of a knife to gently crack them. They should fall off with ease.

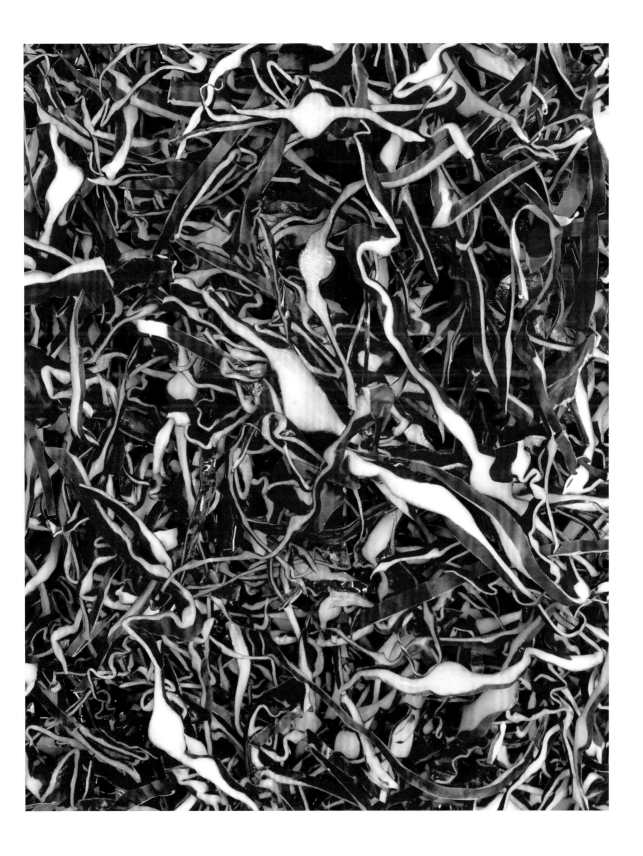

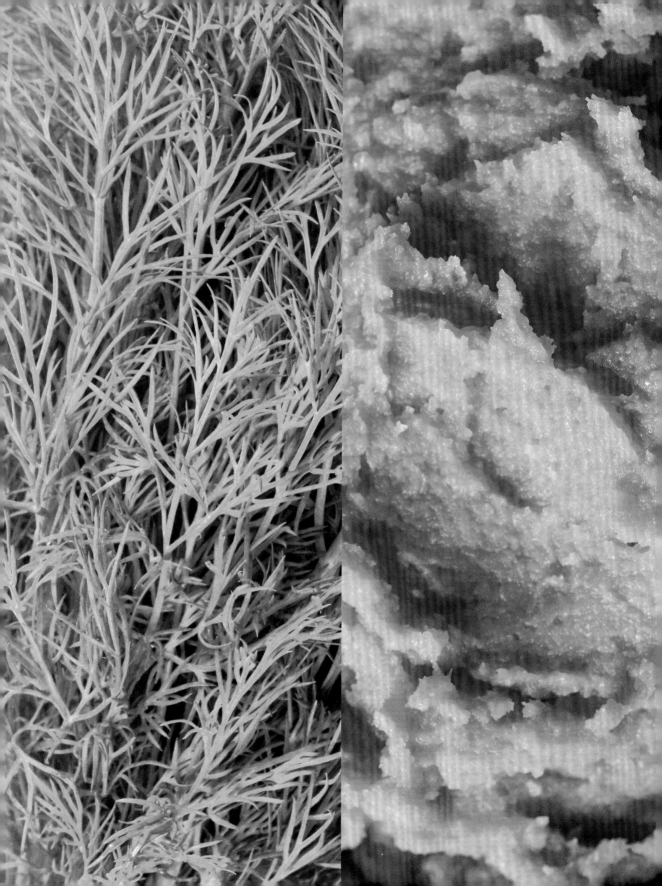

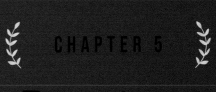

CHAPTER 5

Dressings,
Sauces, and
Condiments

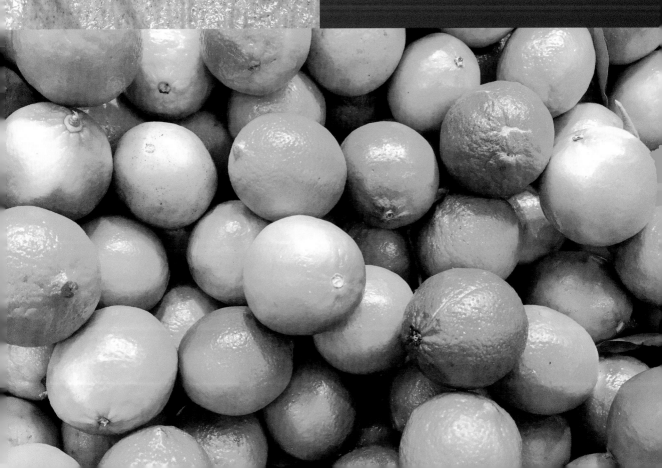

Probiotic Ranch Dressing

I was late to come around to ranch dressing (I know!), but now that I realize what I've been missing, I can't imagine my life without it. This version has all the oniony, garlicky, herb-packed flavors you expect with any ranch, though it gets a lighter spin and dose of probiotics by using milk kefir as the base. Raw garlic and scallions add healthy prebiotics to the mix, too.

MAKES 1 CUP (235 ML)

1 cup (235 ml) live-culture plain milk kefir, preferably whole milk

1 clove garlic, minced

2 scallions, thinly sliced

1 tablespoon (4 g) finely chopped fresh parsley

2 teaspoons finely chopped fresh dill

1 tablespoon (15 ml) freshly squeezed lemon juice

¼ teaspoon kosher salt

¼ teaspoon freshly ground black pepper

1. Place the ingredients in a small, lidded jar and shake well until combined or add to a medium mixing bowl and whisk together.

2. Store the dressing in an airtight container in the refrigerator for up to 4 days. Serve with most any salad or as a dip for vegetables.

Creamy Kefir Poppy Seed Dressing

Poppy seed dressing is a classic, and thanks to its tart flavor with just a touch of sweetness, it toes the line with sweet and savory dishes alike. It can balance the bitter bite of a hearty kale salad or work as the finishing touch that really makes a fruit salad stand out in a crowd.

MAKES ABOUT 1 CUP (235 ML)

½ cup (120 ml) live-culture plain milk kefir, preferably whole milk

3 tablespoons (45 ml) apple cider vinegar

2 tablespoons (40 g) honey, preferably raw

2 tablespoons (28 ml) extra-virgin olive oil

1 teaspoon poppy seeds

½ teaspoon kosher salt

¼ teaspoon freshly ground black pepper

1. Place the ingredients in a small, lidded jar and shake well until combined or add to a medium mixing bowl and whisk together.

2. Store the dressing in an airtight container in the refrigerator for up to 4 days. Serve with sweet or savory salads or appetizers.

Try It Here!

⫸ *Shredded Kale and Radicchio Salad (page 125)*

⫸ *Fruit Salad with Kefir Dressing (page 183)*

Kombucha Vinaigrette

Kombucha isn't just for drinking—this fizzy, fermented tea also makes a great base for a simple vinaigrette, thanks to its vinegar-like taste. Stick with a classic original flavor or give the dressing a touch of something extra by using lemon, ginger, turmeric, or any other flavored kombucha.

MAKES ¾ CUP (175 ML)

¼ cup (60 ml) kombucha

2 tablespoons (28 ml) white wine vinegar

1 tablespoon (15 g) Dijon mustard

1 teaspoon honey, preferably raw

½ teaspoon kosher salt

¼ teaspoon freshly ground black pepper

⅓ cup (80 ml) extra-virgin olive oil

1. Whisk the kombucha, vinegar, mustard, honey, salt, and pepper together in a medium bowl. While whisking, slowly pour in the oil. Continue whisking until emulsified and slightly thickened.

2. Store the vinaigrette in an airtight container in the refrigerator for up to 5 days.

Try It Here!

-»»- *Breakfast Salad with Kombucha Vinaigrette (page 57)*

-»»- *Tricolor Salad with Asparagus and Kombucha Vinaigrette (page 130)*

Orange-Miso Vinaigrette

I have a real thing for a good sweet-and-savory mash-up, and that's a big part of what makes this bright and fruity dressing a favorite. A couple spoonfuls of miso paste add probiotics and lend a salty, umami-rich balance to the sweetness of the orange. The dressing pairs well with almost any salad and makes a great partner to fatty salmon fillets and chicken thighs.

MAKES ¾ CUP (175 ML)

½ cup (120 ml) freshly squeezed orange juice (from 1 large navel orange)

2 tablespoons (28 ml) rice vinegar

2 tablespoons (16 g) white miso paste

1 teaspoon finely grated fresh ginger

1 small clove garlic, minced

¼ teaspoon kosher salt

¼ teaspoon freshly ground black pepper

¼ cup (60 ml) extra-virgin olive oil

1. Add the orange juice, vinegar, miso paste, ginger, garlic, salt, and pepper to a medium bowl. Whisk well until the miso is smooth.

2. Slowly drizzle in the oil while whisking and continue whisking until the vinaigrette is emulsified.

3. Store the vinaigrette in an airtight container in the refrigerator for up to 5 days.

Try It Here!

→ *Citrus-Miso Salmon (page 139)*

→ *Quick Sugar Snap Peas with Orange-Miso Vinaigrette (page 174)*

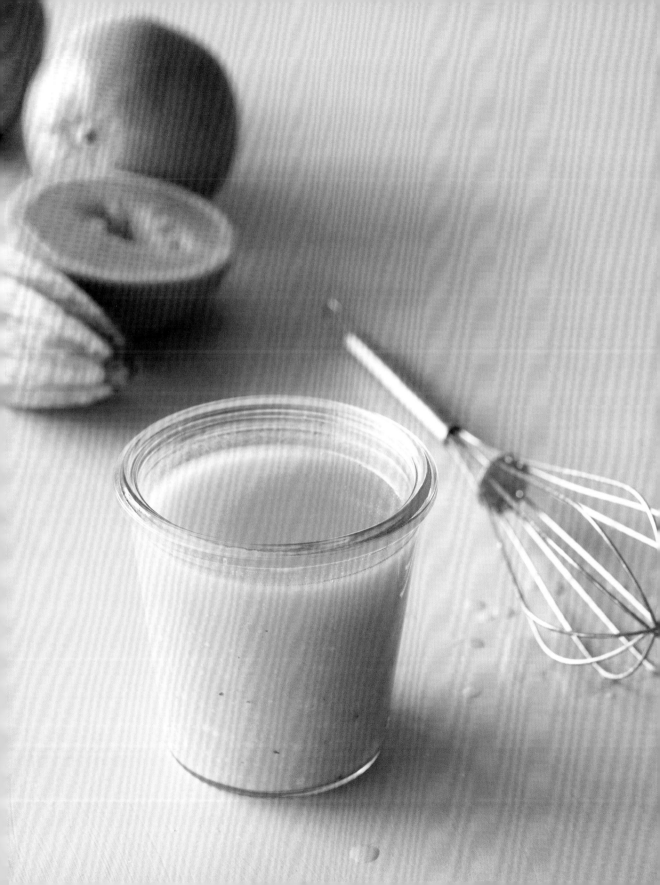

Creamy Honey-Mustard Dressing

Even though it's on the thin side—sitting firmly in dressing territory—this golden-hued, sweet and tangy honey mustard is a great dipping sauce. Beyond drizzling it over salad, it's a wonderful partner to roasted vegetables, chicken, pitas, and wraps.

MAKES ABOUT ¾ CUP (175 ML)

¼ cup (60 ml) live-culture plain milk kefir, preferably whole milk

2 tablespoons (28 ml) extra-virgin olive oil

2 tablespoons (30 g) Dijon mustard

2 tablespoons (40 g) honey, preferably raw

2 tablespoons (28 ml) apple cider vinegar

½ teaspoon kosher salt

¼ teaspoon freshly ground black pepper

1. Place the ingredients in a small, lidded jar and shake well until combined or add to a medium mixing bowl and whisk together.

2. Store the dressing in an airtight container in the refrigerator for up to 4 days.

Try It Here!

→⋙— *Honey-Mustard Chicken Thighs (page 94)*

Creamy Caesar Dressing

Caesar dressing is a lot easier to make at home than you think. Milk kefir works as the base for this creamy, eggless version, which both keeps it light and ups the nutritional value with extra probiotics.

MAKES ABOUT 1 CUP (235 ML)

2 cloves garlic

4 anchovy fillets

¾ cup (175 ml) live-culture plain milk kefir, preferably whole milk

¼ cup (25 g) grated Parmesan

2 tablespoons (28 ml) freshly squeezed lemon juice

1 teaspoon Dijon mustard

1 teaspoon Worcestershire sauce

¼ teaspoon kosher salt

¼ teaspoon freshly ground black pepper

¼ cup (60 ml) extra-virgin olive oil

1. Add the garlic and anchovies to the bowl of a food processor and pulse several times until a thick paste forms. Scrape down the sides of the bowl and add the kefir, Parmesan, lemon juice, mustard, Worcestershire sauce, salt, and pepper. Process continuously until well combined and smooth.

2. With the machine running, gradually pour in the oil and process until emulsified. Store the dressing in an airtight container in the refrigerator for up to 4 days.

Try It Here!

> Smoky Tempeh and Kale Caesar Wraps *(page 110)*

Herbed Yogurt Sauce

I originally planned to share this as a cilantro yogurt sauce (my favorite version of the recipe and the one I make most often). But not everyone loves cilantro, and the truth of the matter is that this creamy sauce works well with just about any fresh herb or combo of herbs you have handy. It blends up thick, just like you'd expect from a sauce, though it can be thinned with a bit of water anytime you want to use it as a salad dressing, which makes it easier to toss with the ingredients.

MAKES JUST OVER ½ CUP (120 ML)

½ cup (115 g) live-culture plain Greek yogurt, preferably whole milk

¼ cup (about 30 g) packed fresh herbs, such as cilantro, parsley, basil, dill, and/or mint

1 clove garlic

Juice of ½ lime

½ teaspoon kosher salt

1 to 2 tablespoons (15 to 28 ml) water, to thin (optional)

1. Add the yogurt, herbs, garlic, lime juice, and salt to a food processor and process continuously, scraping down the sides of the bowl as necessary, until the herbs are broken down and well blended, about 2 minutes. If desired, add water, 1 tablespoon (15 ml) at a time, to thin.

2. Store the vinaigrette in an airtight container in the refrigerator for up to 4 days.

Try It Here!

➤➤ *Herbed Chickpea and Tomato Salad (page 129)*

➤➤ *Miso Brown Rice and Tempeh Buddha Bowls (page 165)*

➤➤ *Harissa-Roasted Carrots with Cilantro-Yogurt Sauce (page 170)*

Miso-Tahini Sauce

I love this sauce just as much for its rich, nutty flavor as for its versatility. It's my secret to instantly upgrading roasted vegetables and stuffed baked potatoes, as well as a go-to for rounding out grain bowls. Use whatever kind of miso paste you have handy. White miso gives the sauce a mellow, subtly sweet flavor, while yellow miso adds a touch more depth, and red miso lends extra-nutty undertones.

MAKES ¾ CUP (175 ML)

¼ cup (60 g) tahini

¼ cup (60 ml) water

2 tablespoons (32 g) miso paste

2 tablespoons (28 ml) rice vinegar

1 teaspoon honey, preferably raw

1 clove garlic, minced

½ teaspoon kosher salt

¼ teaspoon freshly ground black pepper

⅛ teaspoon cayenne pepper

1. Place all the ingredients in a medium bowl and whisk together well until smooth. The sauce will be on the thin side at first and thickens as it sits.

2. Store the sauce in an airtight container in the refrigerator for up to 5 days.

Try It Here!

→ *Charred Broccoli with Miso-Tahini Sauce and Almonds (page 171)*

→ *Probiotic Miso-Tahini Slaw (page 176)*

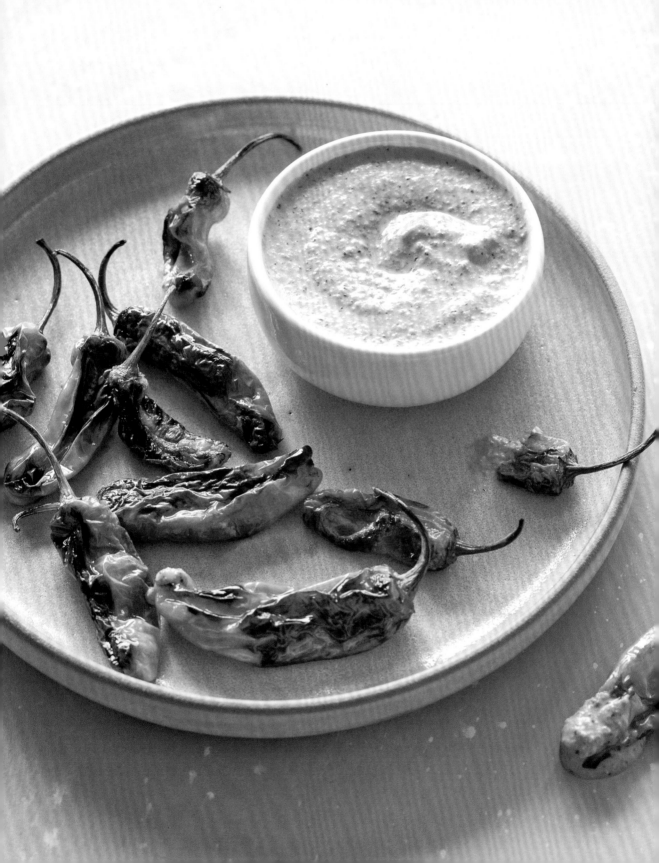

Quick Kimchi Aioli

Aioli has a way of sounding gourmet, yet it's really nothing more than garlicky mayonnaise. This version has the creamy, rich texture you'd expect from classic aioli but gets an extra bright kick from kimchi. It also skips the raw eggs in favor of starting with mayonnaise for ease and simplicity. Drizzle it over steamed or roasted vegetables, use it as a condiment on sandwiches, or try my choice, as a dipping sauce for Blistered Shishitos (page 133).

MAKES 1 CUP (235 ML)

½ cup (50 g) kimchi, drained

2 cloves garlic

½ cup (115 g) mayonnaise

¼ cup (4 g) packed fresh cilantro
   leaves

1. Add the ingredients to the bowl of a food processor and process continuously, scraping down the sides of the bowl as necessary, until well-combined and creamy, 1 to 2 minutes.

2. Store the aioli in an airtight container in the refrigerator for up to 5 days.

Try It Here!

➤ *Blistered Shishitos with Quick Kimchi Aioli (page 133)*

➤ *Salmon Cakes with Quick Kimchi Aioli (page 160)*

Probiotic Kefir Tzatziki

This cool, creamy Mediterranean cucumber dip is typically made with yogurt, leaving it with a thick consistency, though I love to swap in milk kefir. It still comes loaded with probiotics, and the thinner texture makes it even more versatile. In addition to being served as a dip, it makes a great topping for burgers and sandwiches and an excellent choice for drizzling over salads, grain bowls, and fish. If you can't get your hands on preserved lemons, use two teaspoons of freshly squeezed lemon juice instead.

MAKES 1½ CUPS (355 ML)

½ medium English cucumber, peeled and seeded (about ½ cup [70 g])

1 cup (235 ml) live-culture plain milk kefir, preferably whole milk

2 tablespoons (8 g) finely chopped fresh dill

1 clove garlic, minced

1 small preserved lemon, seeded and finely chopped

¼ teaspoon kosher salt

¼ teaspoon freshly ground black pepper

1. Grate the cucumber on the large holes of a box grater, over a clean kitchen towel. Press and drain as much liquid as possible from the cucumbers.

2. Add the cucumber, kefir, dill, garlic, preserved lemon, salt, and pepper to a medium bowl and stir until well combined. Cover and chill for at least 1 hour before serving.

3. Store the tzatziki in an airtight container in the refrigerator for up to 4 days.

Try It Here!

➤ *Chicken Shawarma Pockets with Probiotic Kefir Tzatziki (page 151)*

Dandelion Pesto

If you've been reserving pesto for when you have a bundle of fresh basil, I want you to know that this vibrant sauce can be made with any type of greens you have handy. And that includes dandelion greens, which you're most likely to find in season from late winter through midspring. They can have an aggressive, bitter flavor on their own, so partnering them with a squeeze of lemon juice and umami-rich, salty miso paste mellows the bite to make them shine in this versatile pesto. When eaten raw, dandelion greens are a great source of prebiotics.

MAKES ½ CUP (120 ML)

2 cups (110 g) packed dandelion greens

2 tablespoons (18 g) toasted almonds

2 tablespoons (10 g) grated Parmesan

1 tablespoon (16 g) white miso paste

1 tablespoon (15 ml) lemon juice

1 clove garlic

¼ teaspoon kosher salt

⅓ cup (80 ml) extra-virgin olive oil

1. Add the dandelion greens, almonds, Parmesan, miso paste, lemon juice, garlic, and salt to the bowl of a food processor or blender. Pulse until finely chopped.

2. With the machine running, gradually pour in the oil and process continuously until well combined.

3. Store the pesto in an airtight container in the refrigerator for up to 5 days.

Try It Here!

→»»— *Chilled Sweet Corn Soup with Pesto (page 121)*

→»»— *Farmers Market Pesto Pasta Salad (page 164)*

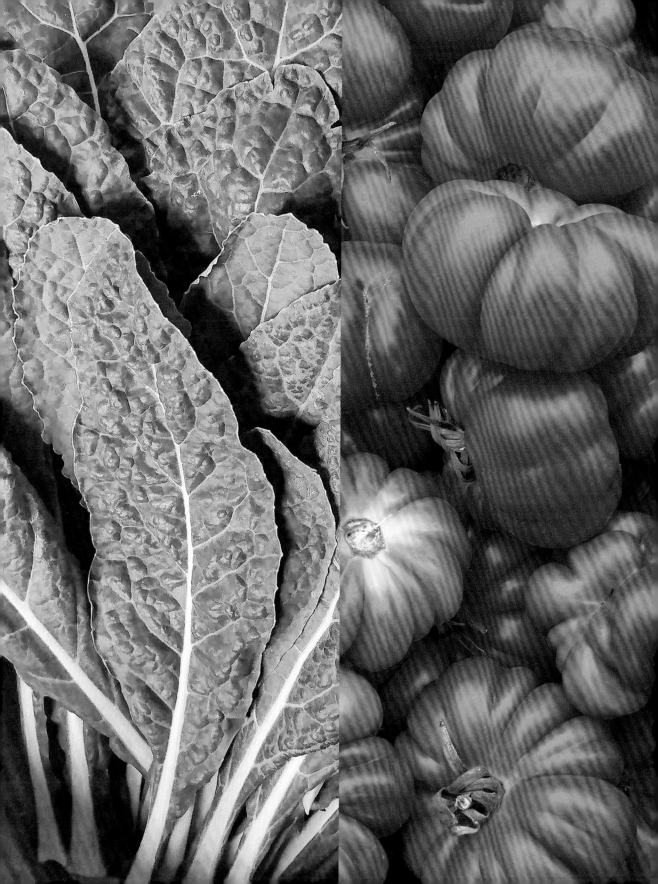

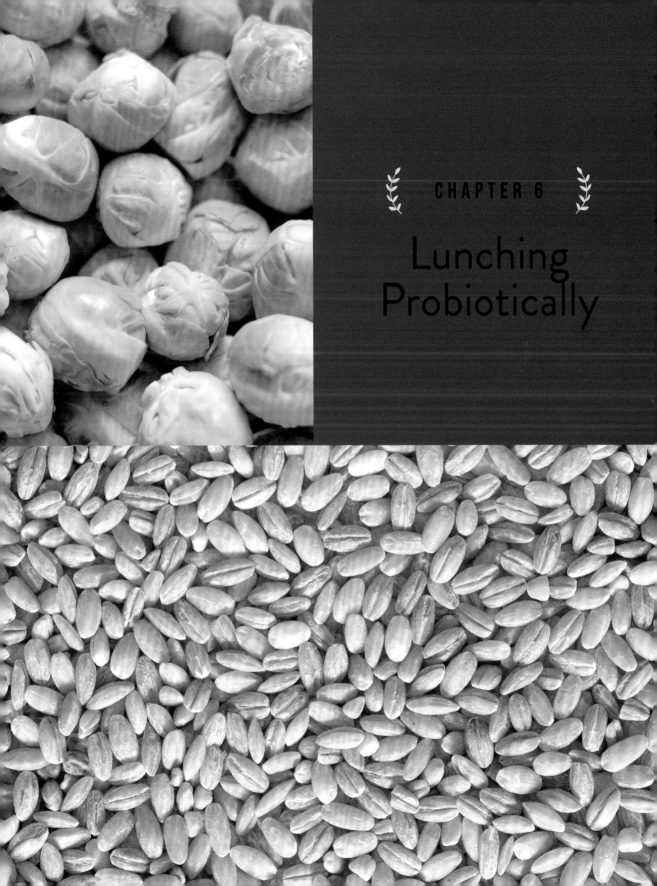

Lunching Probiotically

Kimchi Avocado Toast

Here's some news that's going to make you love avocados even more—they're a great source of prebiotic fiber. Kimchi not only adds probiotics to lunch but is hands down my number-one way to perk up a slice of basic avocado toast. The spicy, tangy flavors are such a fun contrast to the creamy richness of avocado.

SERVES 2

1 avocado, peeled and pitted

1 tablespoon (15 ml) kimchi brine

2 thick-cut slices sourdough bread, lightly toasted

½ cup (50 g) kimchi, drained

SUGGESTED TOPPINGS:
  crumbled nori, toasted sesame seeds, fresh cilantro leaves

1. Add the avocado and kimchi brine to a small bowl and mash together with a fork or the back of a spoon.

2. Spread the mashed avocado over each slice of sourdough. Divide the kimchi between the toasts and top with nori, sesame seeds, or cilantro, as desired.

Almond Butter *and* Miso-Jelly Sandwiches

Nut butter and jelly sandwiches are a classic that I'm convinced will never get old. And I, for one, will never grow out of them. This version blends umami-rich miso paste with the jam for a salty-sweet twist and a touch of probiotics sneaked in. If almond butter isn't your style, go ahead and use peanut butter, cashew butter, or even sunflower seed butter.

MAKES 1 SANDWICH

2 tablespoons (40 g) strawberry jam

2 teaspoons white miso paste

2 tablespoons (32 g) natural almond butter

2 slices multigrain bread

1 tablespoon (6 g) sliced toasted almonds

1. Add the jam and miso paste to a small bowl. Mix well with a fork or spoon until the miso is completely combined and the mixture is smooth.

2. Evenly spread the jam mixture over one slice of the bread and the almond butter over the other slice. Top with sliced almonds and serve.

Kimchi Chicken Salad

The beauty of mild-mannered chicken salad is that it's a total blank slate willing to take on any number of twists and flavors. And the funky bite of gut-friendly kimchi is just the thing to liven up this classic sandwich. If your jar of kimchi contains extra brine, mix a spoonful or two of it into the salad for extra flavor.

SERVES 4

2 pounds (900 g) boneless, skinless chicken breast

1 cup (100 g) kimchi, drained and chopped

½ cup (46 g) toasted sliced almonds

½ cup (115 g) live-culture plain Greek yogurt, preferably whole milk

¼ cup (60 g) mayonnaise

4 scallions, thinly sliced

¼ teaspoon freshly ground black pepper

8 slices sourdough bread

Butter lettuce, for serving (optional)

1. Arrange the chicken in a single layer in a large saucepan. Add cold water to cover the chicken by about 1 inch (2.5 cm). Bring the water to a boil over medium-high heat. Reduce the heat to low and simmer until the chicken is cooked through, 10 to 14 minutes, depending on the thickness. Transfer to a cutting board or large plate and use two forks to shred the chicken. Cool completely.

2. Add the shredded chicken to a large bowl along with the kimchi, almonds, yogurt, mayonnaise, scallions, and pepper and mix together.

3. To serve immediately, divide the chicken salad among the slices of bread and top with lettuce, if desired.

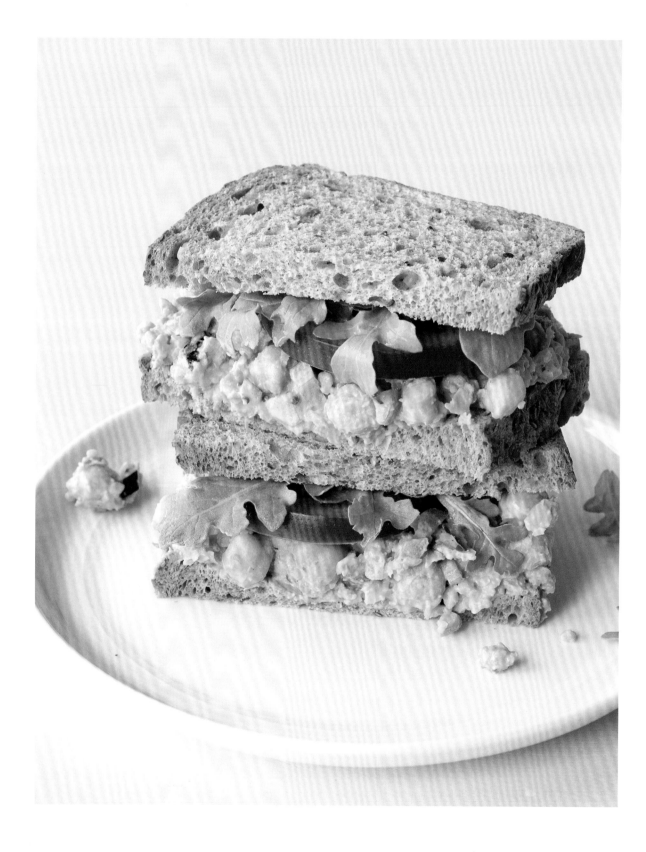

Smashed Chickpea Salad Sandwiches

This vegetarian take on tuna salad celebrates hearty chickpeas as the hero of the sandwich loaded with vegetables. Be sure to use fermented pickles from the refrigerated section of your grocer to take advantage of the probiotic benefits. Also, don't overlook mashing the chickpeas first—it helps these roly-poly beans to stay put on your sandwich.

SERVES 2

1 can (15 ounces, or 425 g) of chickpeas, drained and rinsed, divided

⅓ cup (37 g) shredded carrot

¼ cup (40 g) finely chopped red onion

¼ cup (36 g) chopped fermented pickles

1 celery stalk, finely chopped

¼ cup (60 g) live-culture plain Greek yogurt, preferably whole milk

1 tablespoon (15 ml) apple cider vinegar

2 teaspoons whole grain mustard

½ teaspoon ground turmeric

Kosher salt

Freshly ground black pepper

4 slices multigrain bread

Arugula, for topping

Sliced tomato, for topping

1. Place about half the chickpeas in a large bowl and mash thoroughly with a fork.

2. Add the remaining chickpeas, carrot, onion, pickles, celery, yogurt, vinegar, mustard, turmeric, and pinch of salt and pepper to the bowl and stir to mix together.

3. Divide the chickpea salad evenly between two slices of bread. Top with arugula, sliced tomato, and another slice of bread and serve.

Smoky Tempeh *and* Kale Caesar Wraps

Shredded kale and marinated, smoky lemon tempeh are my trick for giving classic Caesar wraps a fresh twist. Opting for tough kale leaves over Romaine means this salad can be prepped in advance without its going soggy. Do make your own Caesar dressing (it's easier than you think!), which adds an extra probiotic punch to the wraps.

SERVES 4

1 tablespoon (15 ml) freshly squeezed lemon juice

½ teaspoon smoked paprika

¼ teaspoon kosher salt

¼ teaspoon freshly ground black pepper

8 ounces (225 g) tempeh

4 cups (268 g) shredded Tuscan kale (from 1 medium bunch)

¼ cup (20 g) shredded Parmesan

¾ cup (175 ml) Creamy Caesar Dressing (page 95)

2 tablespoons (28 ml) extra-virgin olive oil

4 large flour tortillas

1. Whisk together the lemon juice, paprika, salt, and pepper in a medium bowl until smooth. Cut the tempeh into ¼-inch (6 mm) thick strips. Add to the marinade, gently toss to coat, and let it sit for at least 5 minutes.

2. Meanwhile, add the kale, Parmesan, and dressing to a large bowl. Toss until the leaves are fully coated with the dressing. Set aside.

3. Heat the oil in a large nonstick skillet over medium-high heat until shimmering. Add the tempeh strips and cook until golden brown on all sides, a few minutes per side.

4. To assemble, spoon about one quarter of the kale down the center of a tortilla and top with a few strips of tempeh. Fold the sides of the tortilla over the filling and roll tightly from the bottom up. Repeat with the remaining filling and tortillas. Serve immediately.

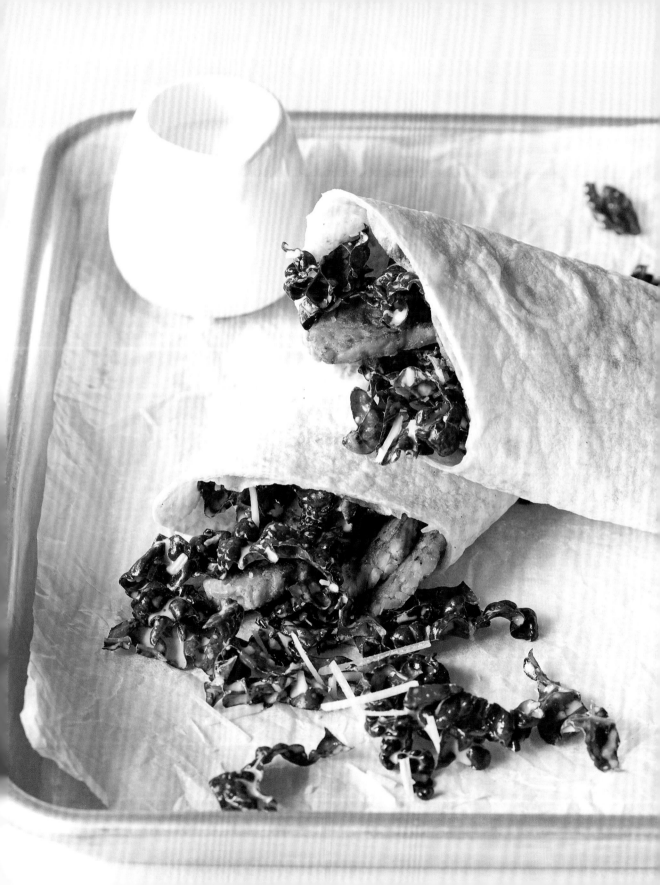

Zesty Grilled Cheese Sandwiches

Mark my word—one of the most delicious ways to get your fill of fermented kraut is stuffed into a melted, gooey grilled cheese sandwich. Gouda (go for an unpasteurized aged version of the cheese, if you can find it, for extra probiotics) is my pick for its top-notch meltability and creamy, nutty taste.

SERVES 2

2 tablespoons (28 g) unsalted butter, room temperature

4 slices sourdough bread

1 tablespoon (15 g) whole grain mustard

2 cups (240 g) grated Gouda (preferably aged), divided

½ cup (120 g) fermented red kraut, drained

½ avocado, peeled, pitted, and thinly sliced

1. Spread the butter over one side of each slice of the bread. Flip over and spread the mustard over the other sides.

2. Heat a large skillet or griddle over medium heat. When hot, add two slices of the bread, butter-side down, to the skillet for the base of the sandwiches. Divide 1 cup (120 g) of the cheese evenly over the two slices of the bread, followed by the kraut and sliced avocado. Sprinkle with the remaining cheese and top with the remaining bread slices, mustard-side down.

3. Cook until the bottom is golden brown and then carefully flip the sandwiches and cook until the other side is lightly browned and the cheese is melted.

4. Transfer to a cutting board, slice the sandwiches in half, and serve immediately.

Heirloom Tomato Sandwich *with* Creamy Roasted Garlic *and* Chive Spread

This is a sandwich to keep on your radar during late summer when those blissfully juicy, sweet heirloom tomatoes roll into the farmers market. There are many ways to make a tomato sandwich, and while not traditional, this one tops the list. The Roasted Garlic and Chive Dip is the perfect highlight for this summer star, and it blends together with a thick and creamy texture, making it just right for a sandwich spread.

SERVES 2

½ cup (120 ml) Creamy Roasted Garlic and Chive Dip (page 132)

4 slices thick-cut sourdough bread

1 ripe heirloom tomato, sliced

½ English cucumber, sliced into rounds

1 avocado, peeled, pitted, and thinly sliced

1. Spread the Creamy Roasted Garlic and Chive Dip on one side of each slice of bread.

2. Top with a layer of sliced tomatoes, followed by sliced cucumbers and sliced avocado. Assemble the sandwiches and serve immediately.

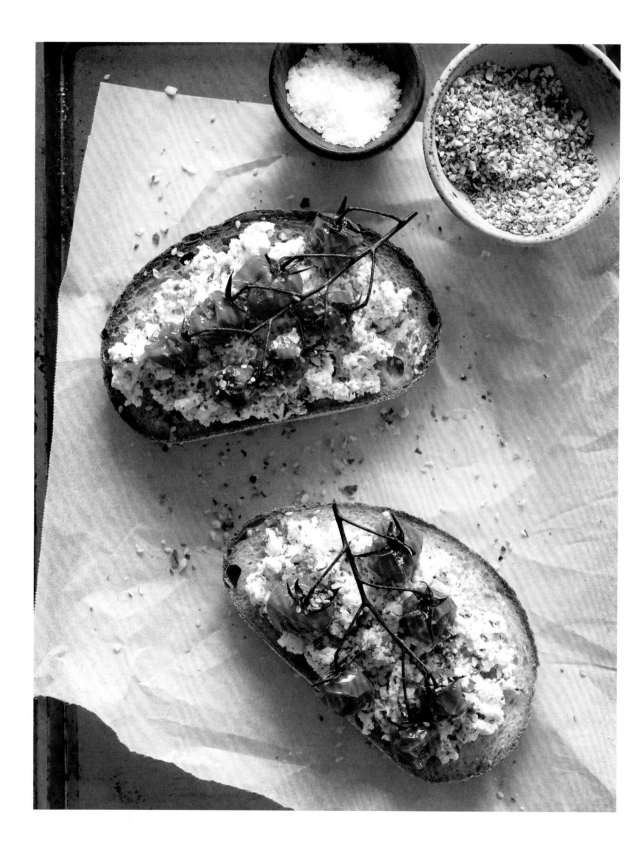

Roasted Tomato Tartine *with* Herbed Cheese

This lunch is a keeper, even in the middle of winter when good tomatoes are nowhere to be found. A quick roast in the oven concentrates their natural sweetness, leaving you with tender, impossibly rich-flavored tomatoes. Inspired by my love for ricotta toast, this quick yet impressive lunch swaps in cultured farmer cheese, which has similar small curds but a slightly drier texture, a tangier taste, and probiotics. Don't skip sprinkling some dukkah over top. It's a Middle Eastern spice blend with herbs, chopped nuts, and seeds, and it rounds out the tartine with a welcome crunch.

SERVES 2

12 cherry tomatoes

1 tablespoon (15 ml) extra-virgin olive oil

2 teaspoons (28 ml) balsamic vinegar

½ cup (120 g) cultured farmer cheese

1 clove garlic, minced

1 tablespoon (3 g) finely chopped fresh basil

1 teaspoon snipped fresh chives

¼ teaspoon kosher salt

2 thick slices sourdough bread, lightly toasted

Flaky sea salt, for topping

Dukkah, for topping

1. Arrange a rack in the middle of the oven and preheat to 425°F (220°C, or gas mark 7).

2. Toss the tomatoes with the oil and vinegar. Place on a parchment-lined rimmed baking sheet. Roast until the tomatoes pop and are lightly browned, 15 to 20 minutes. Set aside to cool.

3. Meanwhile, place the farmer cheese, garlic, basil, chives, and kosher salt in a small bowl. Mix together until light and fluffy.

4. To serve, spread the cheese in an even layer over each slice of the sourdough. Top with roasted tomatoes and sprinkle with flaky salt and dukkah.

Shredded Brussels Sprouts *and* Barley Salad *with* Lemon-Pepper Miso Dressing

My number-one priority when eating salad for lunch (other than its tasting really good!) is that it has to fill me up. To get there, I combine greens and grains, both of which are sources of prebiotics, with beneficial fats from the nuts and olive oil, plus a little cheese for good measure. The dressing has a brightness that's just right for balancing the hearty, slightly bitter greens, and you'll also like the way it soaks into the barley.

SERVES 4

1½ cups (355 ml) water

½ cup (100 g) pearl barley

1 teaspoon kosher salt, divided

¼ cup (60 ml) freshly squeezed lemon juice (from 1 large lemon)

¼ cup (60 ml) extra-virgin olive oil

1 small clove garlic, minced

2 tablespoons (32 g) white miso paste

½ teaspoon freshly ground black pepper

1 pound (455 g) Brussels sprouts, trimmed and shredded

2 cups (110 g) chopped dandelion greens

½ cup (60 g) toasted chopped walnuts

½ cup (40 g) shaved Pecorino cheese

1. Combine the water, barley, and ½ teaspoon of the salt in a medium saucepan. Bring to a boil and then reduce the heat, cover, and simmer until tender and the water has been absorbed, 20 to 25 minutes. Fluff the barley to separate the grains, remove from the heat, and cool completely.

2. Meanwhile, add the lemon juice, oil, garlic, miso paste, the remaining ½ teaspoon of the salt, and the pepper to a small lidded jar. Shake well until combined. Set aside.

3. Add the cooled barley, Brussels sprouts, dandelion greens, walnuts, and Pecorino to a large bowl. Drizzle with the dressing, toss to combine, and serve.

Avocado Egg Salad

Simply by switching out the mayo for yogurt and adding avocado for extra creaminess, classic egg salad instantly gets a boost of probiotics and prebiotics. While the egg salad can certainly be eaten right after it's made, it tastes even better after sitting in the fridge overnight.

SERVES 4

8 hard-boiled eggs, peeled and chopped

1 ripe avocado, peeled and pitted

¼ cup (40 g) finely diced red onion

1 celery stalk, diced

2 tablespoons (8 g) chopped fresh dill

¼ cup (60 g) live-culture plain Greek yogurt, preferably whole milk

1 tablespoon (15 ml) freshly squeezed lemon juice

¼ teaspoon kosher salt

¼ teaspoon freshly ground black pepper

8 slices multigrain bread

SUGGESTED TOPPINGS:
arugula, sliced tomato

1. Add the eggs and avocado to a medium bowl and gently mash together with a fork or the back of a spoon, keeping the mixture a little chunky. Add the onion, celery, dill, yogurt, lemon juice, salt, and pepper and stir well to combine.

2. To serve, divide the egg salad among four slices of the bread. Top each with arugula and tomato, if desired, and place the remaining slices of bread on top of each sandwich. Slice the sandwiches and serve immediately.

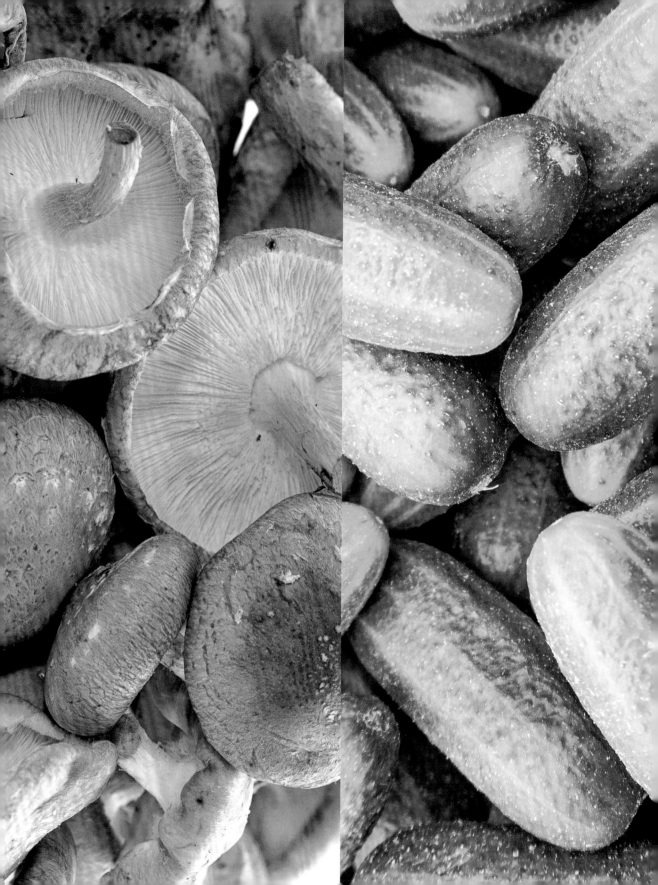

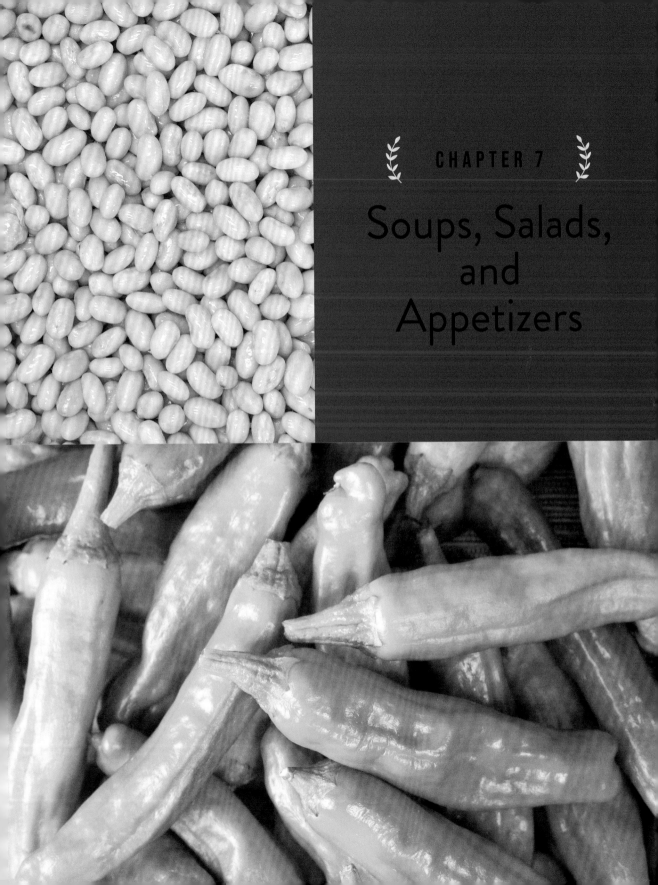

CHAPTER 7

Soups, Salads, and Appetizers

Chilled Sweet Corn Soup with Pesto
121

Restorative Miso Noodle Soup
122

Miso White Bean and Kale Soup with Tempeh Croutons
124

Shredded Kale and Radicchio Salad
125

Smoky Red Lentil Soup with Yogurt
127

Spring Vegetable Panzanella
128

Herbed Chickpea and Tomato Salad
129

Tricolor Salad with Asparagus and Kombucha Vinaigrette
130

Creamy Kale Dip in a Sourdough Bowl
131

Creamy Roasted Garlic and Chive Dip
132

Blistered Shishitos with Quick Kimchi Aioli
133

Pear and Whipped Cheese Crostini
135

Chilled Sweet Corn Soup *with* Pesto

There's no better time to make this refreshing soup than the late summer months when sweet corn is at its peak. The corn is the star of the dish and doesn't need a lot of help to make it shine. Raw dandelion greens are a great source of prebiotics and on their own have a slightly bitter flavor, which works well to balance the natural sweetness of the soup. I love tossing the remainder of the pesto with a simple pasta salad (try the Farmers Market Pesto Pasta Salad on page 164) to round out the dinner.

SERVES 4

2 tablespoons (28 g) unsalted butter

1 small onion, diced

2 cloves garlic, smashed

4 cups (616 g) fresh sweet corn (about 4 ears), cobs reserved

1½ teaspoons kosher salt

¼ teaspoon freshly ground black pepper

3 cups (700 ml) water

½ cup (120 ml) Dandelion Pesto (page 101)

1. Melt the butter in a Dutch oven or large pot over medium heat. Add the onion and garlic and cook, stirring occasionally, until soft, about 5 minutes. Stir in the corn, salt, and pepper. Cook, stirring occasionally, until the corn is soft, about 5 minutes. Pour in the water and add the reserved corn cobs to the pot. Bring to a boil and then reduce the heat and simmer for 10 minutes. Remove and discard the corn cobs.

2. Puree the soup in a blender until smooth, working in batches if necessary.

3. If you prefer a thinner soup, press the soup through a fine-mesh strainer and discard the solids. Otherwise, transfer the soup directly to a large bowl, cover, and chill for at least 2 hours.

4. To serve, divide the soup among four bowls and top with a spoonful of Dandelion Pesto.

Restorative Miso Noodle Soup

Inspired by the calming, nourishing power of classic miso soup, this version gets a hearty upgrade with soba noodles, meaty mushrooms, and spinach. The recipe calls for white miso paste, which has a subtly sweet and mellow flavor, though any variety will work well here. And to maximize its probiotic health benefit, it gets stirred in toward the end of cooking.

SERVES 4

4 ounces (115 g) dried buckwheat soba noodles

1 tablespoon (15 ml) extra-virgin olive oil

1 small onion, diced

1 clove garlic, minced

1 tablespoon (8 g) finely grated fresh ginger

½ teaspoon kosher salt

¼ teaspoon freshly ground black pepper

4 cups (946 ml) low-sodium chicken or vegetable broth

1 tablespoon (15 ml) soy sauce or tamari

¼ cup (64 g) white miso paste

6 ounces (170 g) silken tofu, cut into ½-inch (1.3 cm) cubes

2 ounces (55 g) shiitake mushrooms, thinly sliced

2 cups (60 g) packed baby spinach

2 scallions, thinly sliced

1. Cook the soba noodles in a Dutch oven or large pot according to the package instructions. Drain and rinse with cold water to remove the excess starch. Set aside. Wipe the pot clean.

2. In the same pot, heat the oil over medium heat until shimmering. Add the onion, garlic, ginger, salt, and pepper and cook, stirring occasionally, until soft, about 3 minutes. Pour in the broth and soy sauce. Bring to a boil and then reduce the heat and simmer for 10 minutes.

3. Add the miso paste and whisk until completely dissolved. Add the tofu, mushrooms, and spinach and simmer for 5 minutes more. Stir in the cooked soba noodles and scallions. Serve immediately.

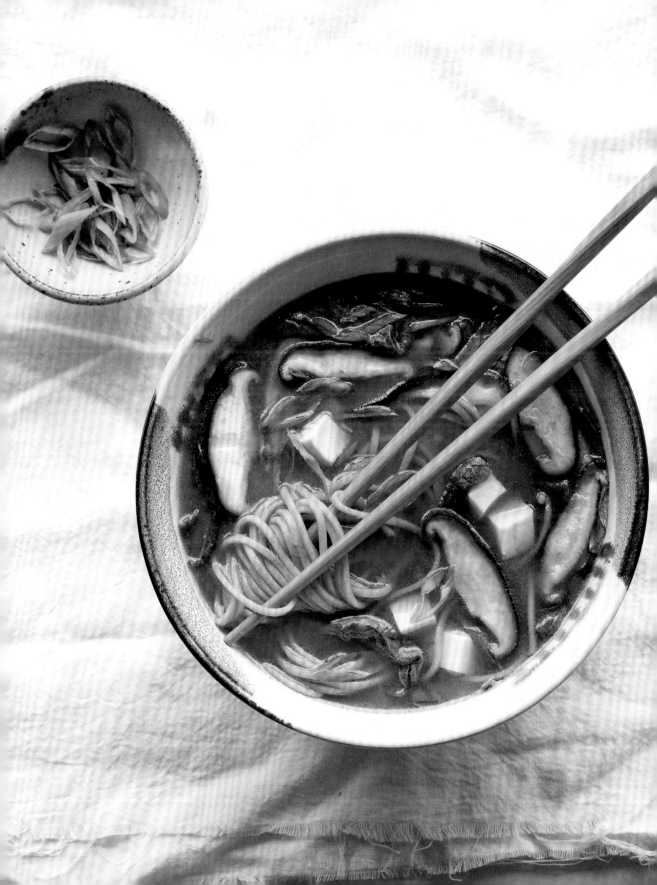

Miso White Bean *and* Kale Soup *with* Tempeh Croutons

Because probiotics lose their effectiveness the more they're exposed to heat, this recipe gives the tempeh croutons just a quick, gentle sear and waits until nearly the end of cooking to blend the miso paste into the broth to maximize the nutritional benefit.

SERVES 4

4 tablespoons (60 ml) extra-virgin olive oil, divided

1 medium onion, diced

1 large carrot, peeled and diced

2 celery ribs, diced

2 cloves garlic, minced

1½ teaspoons kosher salt

¼ teaspoon freshly ground black pepper

¼ teaspoon red pepper flakes

2 cans (15 ounces, or 425 g each) of cannellini beans, drained and rinsed

4 cups (946 ml) low-sodium vegetable or chicken broth

¼ cup (64 g) white or yellow miso paste

3 cups (201 g) chopped Tuscan kale leaves (about 1 small bunch)

1 package (8-ounce or 225 g) of tempeh, cut into ½-inch (1.3 cm) cubes

1. Heat 2 tablespoons (28 ml) of the oil in a Dutch oven or large pot over medium heat until shimmering. Add the onion, carrot, and celery and cook, stirring occasionally, until soft, about 5 minutes. Stir in the garlic, salt, black pepper, and red pepper flakes and cook for 1 minute more.

2. Add the beans and broth to the pot. Bring the soup to a boil and then reduce the heat to a simmer. Ladle about 2 cups (475 ml) of the broth and beans to a blender. Add the miso paste and blend on low speed until smooth. (Alternatively, use an immersion blender to blend the soup slightly in the pot.) Return the puree to the pot along with the kale. Bring the soup to a simmer and cook until the kale is wilted, about 10 minutes. Meanwhile, prepare the tempeh croutons.

3. Heat the remaining 2 tablespoons (28 ml) of oil in a large nonstick skillet over medium-high heat. Add the tempeh cubes and cook, flipping occasionally, until all sides are golden brown and crispy, about 5 minutes.

4. To serve, divide the soup among four bowls and top with the tempeh croutons.

Shredded Kale *and* Radicchio Salad

This is an everyday salad you'll find me making for lunches or as a side for dinner almost every week. In addition to having the extra helping of vegetables, it's my way of working prebiotics (here, the radicchio and avocado) into mealtime on a regular basis. You can't go wrong with any dressing you drizzle over top, but the Creamy Kefir Poppy Seed Dressing, which adds a dose of probiotics, is always my favorite with this mix.

SERVES 4

1 large bunch Tuscan kale, leaves thinly shredded

1 head radicchio, thinly shredded

1 cup (110 g) shredded carrot

2 Persian cucumbers, sliced

1 watermelon radish, thinly sliced

1 avocado, peeled, pitted, and chopped

½ cup (75 g) feta cheese, crumbled

¼ cup (25 g) toasted almonds, chopped

⅓ to ½ cup (80 to 120 ml) Creamy Kefir Poppy Seed Dressing (page 90)

1. Add the kale, radicchio, carrot, cucumbers, radish, avocado, feta, and almonds to a large bowl.

2. Drizzle ⅓ cup (80 ml) of the Creamy Kefir Poppy Seed Dressing around the edges of the bowl and toss to combine. Add more dressing as desired and serve.

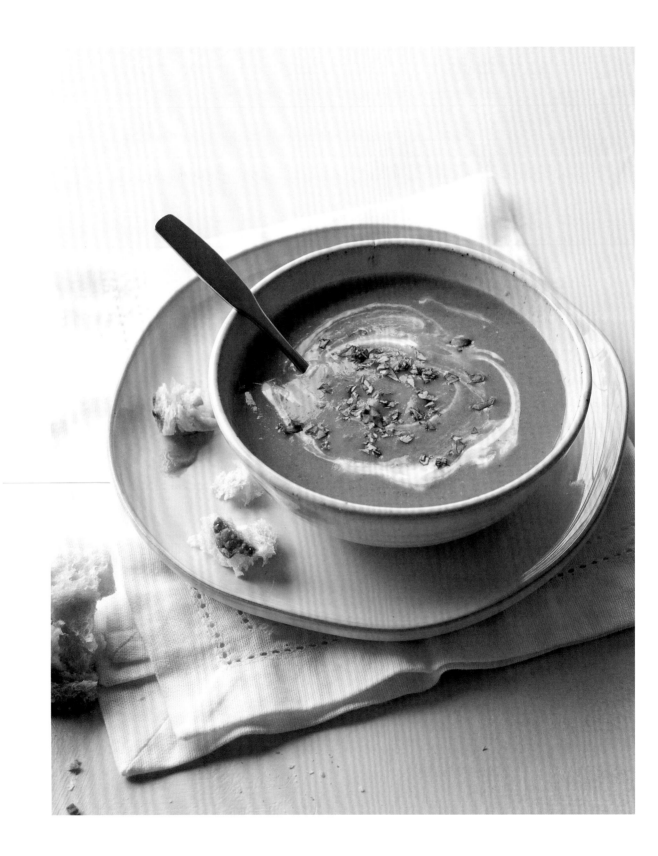

Smoky Red Lentil Soup *with* Yogurt

There are big and small ways to work probiotics into your day, and while this is a relatively small one, it's also incredibly easy. Creamy Greek yogurt is a wonderful addition to round out a bowl of soup. The yogurt is stirred in at the very end to minimize its exposure to heat and maximize the nutritional benefit of probiotics. I also recommend adding a generous dollop on top for serving. It adds just the right balance to the soup's thick and hearty texture and notes of spice.

SERVES 4 TO 6

3 tablespoons (45 ml) extra-virgin olive oil

1 medium onion, diced

2 medium carrots, peeled and diced

2 celery ribs, diced

3 cloves garlic, minced

1 tablespoon (7 g) smoked paprika

2 teaspoons ground cumin

2 teaspoons kosher salt

1 teaspoon ground turmeric

½ teaspoon freshly ground black pepper

1½ cups (288 g) red lentils

6 cups (1.4 L) low-sodium vegetable broth

½ cup (115 g) live-culture plain Greek yogurt, preferably whole milk, plus more for topping

Chopped fresh cilantro, for topping

1. Heat the oil in a Dutch oven or large pot over medium heat until shimmering. Add the onion, carrots, celery, and garlic and cook, stirring occasionally, until soft, 5 to 8 minutes. Stir in the paprika, cumin, salt, turmeric, and pepper and cook for 1 minute more. Add the lentils and broth and bring the soup to a boil. Reduce the heat and simmer until the lentils are tender, about 20 minutes.

2. Remove the soup from the heat and cool slightly. Puree the soup with an immersion blender or in a traditional blender, working in batches, if necessary. Stir in the yogurt.

3. To serve, divide the soup among four to six bowls and top with an additional dollop of yogurt and some chopped cilantro.

Spring Vegetable Panzanella

Panzanella is a Tuscan summer salad typically made with tomatoes and stale bread cubes soaked in a vinegary dressing. And while skewing from the traditional, it's easily adapted to almost any seasonal vegetables currently available. Just don't forget the cubes of crunchy bread, which can be dried out in the oven when you don't have a stale loaf handy. This springtime version of panzanella makes asparagus the star, which, along with raw red onions and garlic, is a good source of prebiotics. While thick or thin asparagus spears work nicely, I think the milder thin ones are the better choice for uncooked dishes.

SERVES 4 TO 6

2 cups (100 g) sourdough bread cubes

¼ cup (60 ml) freshly squeezed lemon juice

¼ cup (60 ml) extra-virgin olive oil

1 tablespoon (16 g) white miso paste

1 teaspoon Dijon mustard

1 clove garlic, minced

½ teaspoon kosher salt

¼ teaspoon freshly ground black pepper

½ small red onion, thinly sliced

1 bundle thin asparagus, trimmed and cut into 2-inch (5 cm) pieces

1 small bunch radishes, quartered

½ fennel bulb, thinly sliced

½ cup (75 g) feta cheese, crumbled

1. Arrange a rack in the middle of the oven and preheat to 300°F (150°C, or gas mark 2).

2. Place the bread cubes on a rimmed baking sheet in a single layer. Bake until dried out and crisp on the outside, about 20 minutes, tossing once halfway through. Cool completely.

3. Meanwhile, whisk together the lemon juice, olive oil, miso paste, mustard, garlic, salt, and pepper in a large bowl until emulsified. Add the onion, stir to coat, and let it sit until the bread cubes are cooled.

4. Add the bread cubes, asparagus, radishes, fennel, and feta to the bowl with the dressing and onions and toss to combine. Serve immediately.

Cooking Tip!

To mellow the sharp and sometimes overwhelming bite of sliced or chopped raw onion, soak it in dressing for several minutes before tossing the rest of your salad ingredients into the bowl.

Herbed Chickpea *and* Tomato Salad

The dressing for this Mediterranean-inspired bean and vegetable salad is wonderfully versatile and can be made with any type of fresh herbs you have on hand (see page 96). For this salad, I think parsley, basil, and dill work well—or even a combination of those herbs. I also recommend thinning the sauce with a tablespoon or two (15 to 28 ml) of water to make it easier to toss together.

SERVES 4

2 cans (15-ounce or 425 g each) of chickpeas, drained and rinsed (or 3 cups [492 g] cooked)

2 cups (360 g) grape tomatoes, halved

3 Persian cucumbers, chopped

½ small red onion, chopped

½ cup (90 g) chopped roasted red peppers

½ cup (75 g) feta cheese, crumbled

½ cup (120 ml) Herbed Yogurt Sauce (page 96)

1. Add the chickpeas, tomatoes, cucumbers, onion, red peppers, and feta to a large bowl.

2. Drizzle ¼ cup (60 ml) of the Herbed Yogurt Sauce around the bowl and toss to combine. Mix in additional dressing, as desired, and serve.

Tricolor Salad *with* Asparagus *and* Kombucha Vinaigrette

Whenever I feel like I'm in a salad rut, this simple and colorful mixture snaps me out of it every time. And, as a bonus, this salad is all about the prebiotics. Instead of my standard lettuce or spinach base, it starts with spicy arugula, endive, and radicchio. The latter two, along with asparagus and red onion, also deliver more prebiotics to your plate. Stick with thin asparagus for this salad, which has a mellower, milder, slightly sweeter flavor than their thick, sometimes grassy counterpart.

SERVES 4

1 endive, shredded

1 small head radicchio, thinly shredded

2 cups (40 g) packed arugula

½ bundle thin asparagus, trimmed and cut into 2-inch (5 cm) pieces

½ cup (58 g) red onion, thinly sliced

¾ cup (175 g) Kombucha Vinaigrette (page 91)

½ cup (40 g) shaved Parmesan

¼ cup (35 g) toasted pine nuts

1. Combine the endive, radicchio, arugula, asparagus, and red onion in a large bowl.

2. Drizzle half of the Kombucha Vinaigrette around the edge of the bowl and toss to coat. Top the salad with the shaved Parmesan and pine nuts and additional vinaigrette, as desired, and serve.

Creamy Kale Dip *in a* Sourdough Bowl

If this probiotic-rich dip reminds you of classic spinach dip—you know, the kind you grew up with, served in a hollowed-out bread bowl—you wouldn't be wrong. This is a lightened-up twist on the timeless party favorite, mixed with sautéed hearty kale and a generous dose of probiotics. Kefir is mixed with the Greek yogurt base, to thin the dip just a touch and add a little extra zing. I recommend the whole-milk version of each, which gives the dip a richer, creamier flavor and thicker texture.

MAKES ABOUT 2½ CUPS (570 ML)

1 tablespoon (15 ml) extra-virgin olive oil

2 cups (134 g) Tuscan kale leaves (about 1 small bunch), finely chopped

1 shallot, finely chopped

1 clove garlic, minced

1½ cups (345 g) live-culture plain Greek yogurt, preferably whole milk

½ cup (120 ml) live-culture plain milk kefir, preferably whole milk

½ teaspoon sweet paprika

½ teaspoon kosher salt

¼ teaspoon freshly ground black pepper

1 round loaf sourdough (8 ounces, or 225 g)

1. Heat the oil in a large skillet over medium heat until shimmering. Add the kale, shallot, and garlic and cook, stirring frequently, until the kale is wilted and the shallot is tender, about 5 minutes. Remove from the heat and cool completely.

2. Add the cooled kale mixture, yogurt, kefir, paprika, salt, and pepper to a medium bowl and stir well to combine. Chill for at least 1 hour before serving.

3. Hollow out the sourdough loaf, leaving a 2-inch (5 cm) wall around the edge. Cut the interior of the bread into bite-size pieces and use for serving. Spoon the dip into the bread bowl and serve, along with the pieces of bread.

Creamy Roasted Garlic *and* Chive Dip

Before you question using a full head of garlic for this creamy dip, I assure you that the measurements are just right. Roasting transforms garlic into something magical, mellowing its once sharp, powerful bite into a rich, full-flavored taste that is completely luxurious. The dip blends up smooth and somewhat thick, which also makes it an ideal spread for sandwiches, wraps, and burgers. You can get a head start by roasting the garlic a day in advance and then storing it in the fridge until you're ready to blend the dip together.

MAKES 1½ CUPS (355 ML)

1 head garlic

1 teaspoon extra-virgin olive oil

1 cup (225 g) cultured cottage cheese

1 cup (230 g) live-culture plain Greek yogurt, preferably whole milk

½ teaspoon kosher salt

¼ teaspoon freshly ground black pepper

¼ cup (12 g) snipped chives

1. Arrange a rack in the middle of the oven and preheat to 400°F (200°C, or gas mark 6).

2. Peel away and discard the papery outer layers of the head of garlic. Leaving the head intact, trim off about ¼ inch (6 mm) from the top of the head to expose the cloves. Drizzle the oil over the top of the garlic. Wrap in foil and roast for 45 minutes. Unwrap the garlic and cool completely.

3. Once cool, add the garlic, cottage cheese, yogurt, salt, and pepper to a food processor. Process continuously until smooth and well combined, about 30 seconds. Scrape down the sides of the bowl, if necessary, and add the chives. Pulse several times until the chives are just combined.

4. Serve the dip with veggies, crackers, pita, or fresh bread.

Try It Here!

- *Loaded Portobello Burgers (page 146)*
- *Heirloom Tomato Sandwiches with Creamy Roasted Garlic and Chive Dip (page 113)*

Blistered Shishitos *with* Quick Kimchi Aioli

The very best way to eat shishito peppers is with their skins gently charred, the flesh having roasted just long enough to become tender without getting too soft. Eating shishitos is like a game of roulette. For the most part these peppers aren't spicy, but in every bunch there are always a few that will surprise your taste buds with a burst of heat. I recommend serving them with a creamy Quick Kimchi Aioli, which complements the char and balances out any spice that comes your way.

Midsummer through fall is when shishito peppers are at their prime and readily available at farmers markets, though you'll have luck finding them in grocery stores throughout the year.

SERVES 4

1 tablespoon (15 ml) extra-virgin olive oil

12 ounces (340 g) shishito peppers (about 32 peppers)

Flaky salt

1 cup (235 ml) Quick Kimchi Aioli (page 99)

1. Heat the oil in a cast-iron skillet over medium-high heat until shimmering. Add the peppers to the skillet in a single layer and cook undisturbed until the bottoms begin to char, about 3 minutes. Cook, tossing occasionally, until lightly charred and blistered all over, 3 to 4 minutes more.

2. Transfer the peppers to a large plate or platter and sprinkle with flaky salt. Serve with the Quick Kimchi Aioli for dipping.

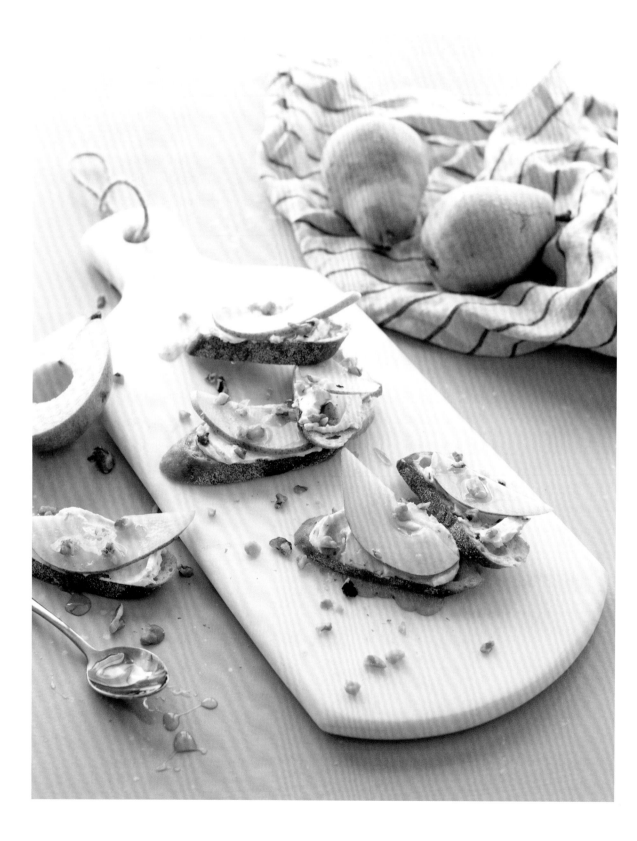

Pear *and* Whipped Cheese Crostini

Crostini is a guaranteed crowd-pleaser. And with a mix of savory, sweet, nutty flavors and creamy, crunchy textures, this one does not disappoint. On its own, probiotic-rich farmer cheese is fairly bland and far more dry than it is creamy. But whip it together with a little bit of goat cheese, fresh herbs, and garlic, and it's nothing short of luxurious. The toast rounds can be made a day in advance, as can the whipped cheese spread. Store the cheese in the refrigerator and let it sit at room temperature for about 10 minutes before assembling the crostini.

MAKES ABOUT 20 CROSTINI

1 baguette, sliced on a bias into ¼-inch (6 mm) thick pieces

1 tablespoon (15 ml) extra-virgin olive oil

1 cup (80 g) cultured farmer cheese, room temperature

2 ounces (55 g) goat cheese, room temperature

1 clove garlic, minced

¼ teaspoon kosher salt

Pinch freshly ground black pepper

½ teaspoon dried thyme

2 Anjou pears, cored and thinly sliced

¼ cup (30 g) chopped toasted walnuts

Honey, preferably raw, for drizzling

1. Arrange a rack in the middle of the oven and preheat to 300°F (150°C, or gas mark 2). Lightly brush the baguette slices with the oil and place in a single layer on a rimmed baking sheet. Bake until lightly browned and crisp around the edges, about 8 minutes. Remove from the oven and cool completely.

2. Meanwhile, add the farmer cheese, goat cheese, garlic, salt, and pepper to the bowl of a food processor and process continuously until the mixture is light and fluffy, about 1 minute. Add the thyme and pulse to combine.

3. To assemble, spread a thick layer of the whipped cheese over each slice of bread, top with a slice of pear, walnuts, and a drizzle of honey. Serve at room temperature.

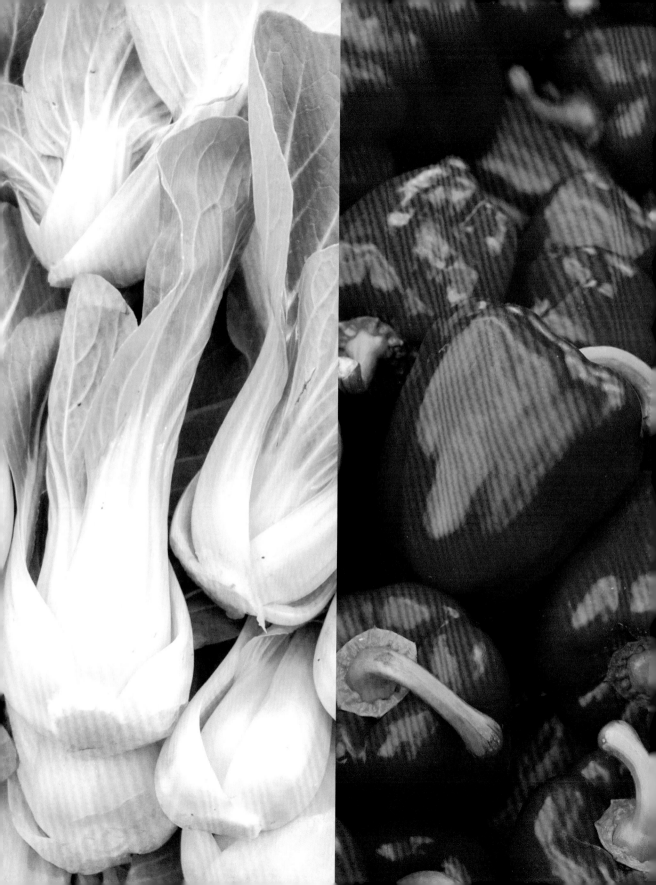

Main Dishes

Citrus-Miso Salmon

A simple sweet-and-savory citrus vinaigrette is my secret to instantly transforming a basic salmon fillet into a fast yet elegant dinner. Here the Orange-Miso Vinaigrette pulls double duty as a marinade and a sauce for serving.

SERVES 4

¾ cup (175 ml) Orange-Miso Vinaigrette (page 92), divided

4 skin-on salmon fillets (6-ounces, or 170 g)

Kosher salt

Freshly ground black pepper

2 scallions, thinly sliced

1. Add ¼ cup (60 ml) of the Orange-Miso Vinaigrette to a wide, shallow container to marinate the salmon. Place the salmon fillets in the container skin-side up. Cover and marinate the salmon in the refrigerator for at least 10 minutes.

2. Arrange an oven rack about 6 inches (15 cm) below the broiler and set the oven to broil (grill).

3. Place the salmon on a foil-lined rimmed baking sheet, skin-side down, season with salt and pepper, and discard the marinade. Broil until the salmon flakes easily and is cooked through, 6 to 8 minutes depending on the thickness.

4. To serve, divide the salmon among four plates, drizzle each fillet with a couple of spoonfuls of the remaining Orange-Miso Vinaigrette, and top with the scallions.

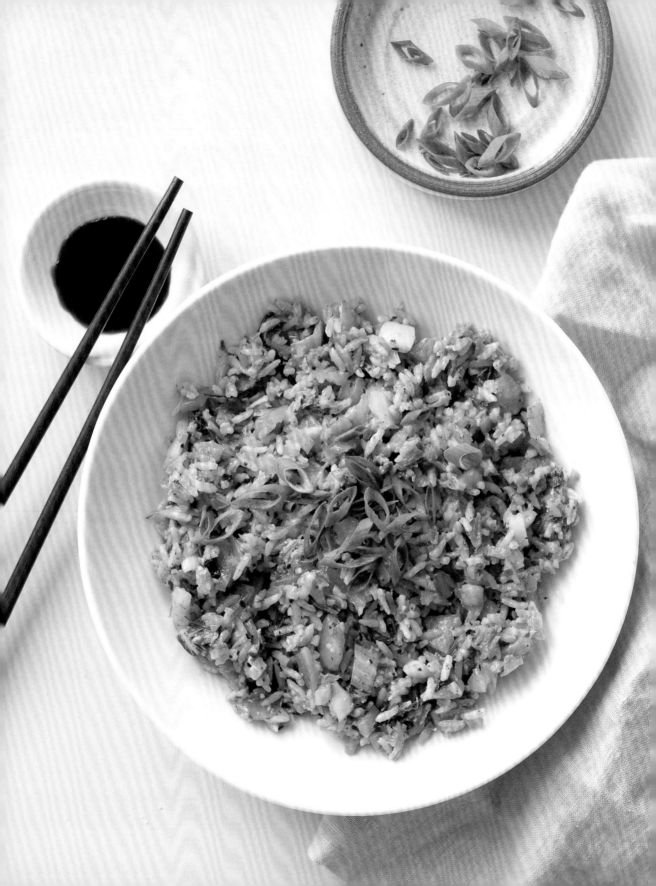

Kimchi Fried Rice

As with any fried rice, this gut-friendly version comes together fast, so you'll want to have all the ingredients at the ready when you step up to the stove. Kimchi brings a flavorful punch and kicks things up with a little heat.

SERVES 4

2 tablespoons (28 ml) canola or vegetable oil, divided

1 small onion, diced

2 cloves garlic, minced

3 bunches baby bok choy, chopped

1½ cups (150 g) kimchi, drained and chopped, divided

3 cups (474 g) cooked long-grain white rice, preferably day-old

3 scallions, thinly sliced, plus more for serving

½ teaspoon kosher salt

2 large eggs, beaten

2 tablespoons (28 ml) soy sauce or tamari

1. Heat 1 tablespoon (15 ml) of the oil in a wok or large nonstick skillet over medium-high heat until shimmering. Add the onion and garlic and stir-fry for 1 minute. Add the bok choy and ½ cup (50 g) of the kimchi and stir-fry until heated through, about 30 seconds.

2. Add the remaining 1 tablespoon (15 ml) of oil and swirl around the pan. Add the rice, scallions, and salt and stir-fry for 2 minutes.

3. Push the rice to the outer edges of the pan, creating a well at the center. Pour the eggs into the center of the pan. Use a spatula to scramble the eggs and once they begin to set, mix them together with the rice. Remove the pan from the heat. Add the remaining 1 cup (100 g) of kimchi and the soy sauce and stir to combine. Top with extra sliced scallions and serve immediately.

Fish Tacos *with* Kefir-Avocado Crema

A few slices of avocado and a generous forkful of quick-pickled vegetables used to be my standard way to top off any and all types of fish tacos. That was, until I realized that with a couple small changes I could seamlessly incorporate probiotics into dinner. Fermented kraut makes an ideal stand-in for pickled vegetables, and instead of slices, the avocado gets blitzed with probiotic-rich milk kefir and a squeeze of lime for a quick and creamy crema.

SERVES 4 (MAKES 8 TACOS)

2 teaspoons chili powder

1¼ teaspoons kosher salt, divided

½ teaspoon garlic powder

¼ teaspoon freshly ground black pepper

1 pound (455 g) skinless, thin, mild white fish fillets, such as tilapia, snapper, flounder, or catfish

1 tablespoon (15 ml) extra-virgin olive oil

1 ripe avocado, peeled and pitted

½ cup (120 ml) live-culture plain milk kefir, preferably whole milk

Juice of 1 lime

8 corn tortillas, (6 inches, or 15 cm each), warmed

1 cup (240 g) fermented red cabbage kraut

Fresh cilantro leaves, for topping

1. Arrange a rack in the middle of the oven and preheat to 400°F (200°C, or gas mark 6).

2. Mix together the chili powder, 1 teaspoon of the salt, the garlic powder, and pepper in a small bowl. Lightly brush the fish with the oil on both sides, coat with the spice blend, and place on a rimmed baking sheet. Bake until cooked through, 6 to 8 minutes, depending on the thickness. Once cool enough to handle, slice the fish into thin strips. Meanwhile, prepare the crema.

3. Add the avocado, kefir, lime juice, and remaining ¼ teaspoon of salt to a food processor and process continuously until smooth. Alternatively, the crema can be blended together using an immersion blender.

4. To assemble, divide the fish among the tortillas, top with kraut, Kefir-Avocado Crema, and fresh cilantro. Serve immediately.

Tempeh Summer Rolls

If you've never made summer rolls before, they might make you feel a little bit intimidated. Here's the thing—it's not nearly as tricky as it looks. You'll get the hang of it after a roll or two, and it will keep getting easier from there. Start by whisking together a sauce (with a hint of prebiotics and probiotics mixed in) that serves as both a marinade for the tempeh and a dipping sauce for the rolls. While the tempeh needs only a few minutes to soak up flavor from the marinade, I like to let it sit while I prep the vegetables.

SERVES 4

FOR THE MARINADE AND DIPPING SAUCE:

¼ cup (60 ml) rice vinegar

2 tablespoons (28 ml) freshly squeezed lime juice

1 tablespoon (20 g) honey, preferably raw

1 tablespoon (16 g) white or yellow miso paste

1 teaspoon soy sauce or tamari

1 teaspoon Asian fish sauce

8 ounces (225 g) tempeh, cut into thin strips

1 tablespoon (15 ml) canola or vegetable oil

FOR THE FILLING:

8 rice paper sheets

24 fresh basil or mint leaves

1 medium carrot, peeled and julienned

1 small seedless cucumber, julienned

1 small red bell pepper, thinly sliced

2 scallions, julienned

1 medium avocado, peeled, pitted, and thinly sliced

1. In a small bowl, whisk together the rice vinegar, lime juice, honey, miso paste, soy sauce, and fish sauce.

2. Add the tempeh to a medium bowl and spoon 3 tablespoons (45 ml) of the sauce over top. Marinate the tempeh for at least 5 minutes. Set aside the remainder of the sauce.

3. Heat the oil in a large nonstick skillet over medium-high heat until shimmering. Add the tempeh strips and cook until golden brown all over, about 2 minutes per side.

4. Fill a wide, shallow bowl or skillet with warm water. Add 1 sheet of rice paper and soak until pliable, about 30 seconds. Remove from the water and lie flat on a damp kitchen towel.

5. To assemble, place several basil or mint leaves down the length of the rice paper wrapper, slightly off-center and leaving ½ inch (1.3 cm) of wrapper at the top and bottom. Top with a few strips of tempeh, followed by an even amount of carrot, cucumber, bell pepper, scallions, and two slices of avocado. Fold the top and bottom of the wrapper over the filling. Fold one side of the wrapper over the filling and roll tightly until it's closed. Place on a plate, seam-side down, and cover with a damp towel. Repeat with the remaining rolls. Serve immediately.

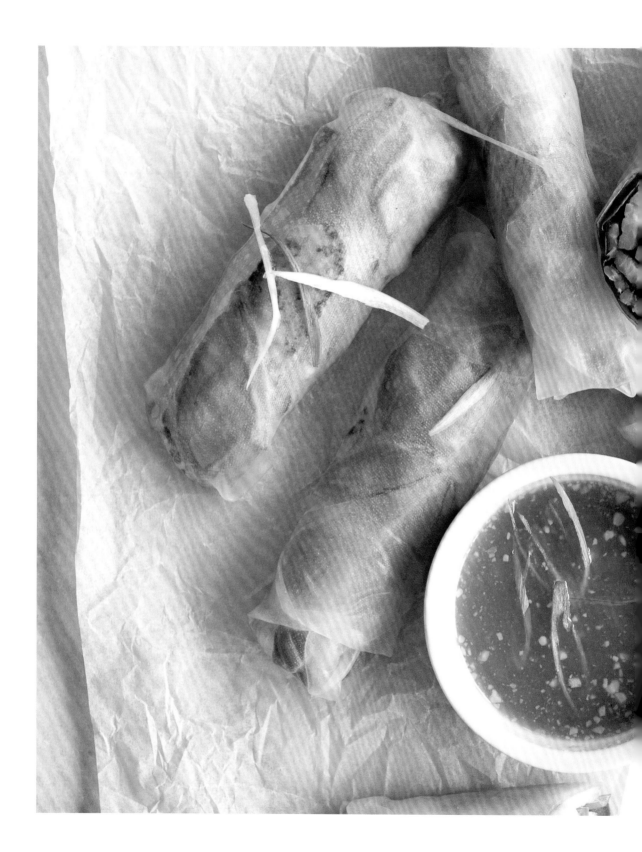

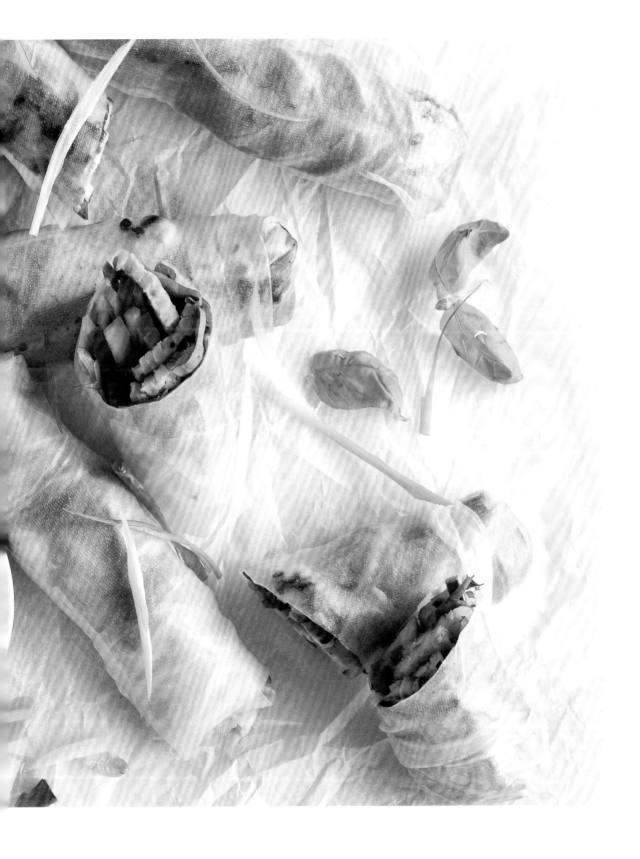

Loaded Portobello Burgers

Between the rich and garlicky spread, some spicy kraut, and a generous scoop of prebiotic-rich avocado layered around a meaty roasted portobello, this recipe will forever change the way you think about veggie burgers.

SERVES 4

4 large portobello mushrooms, stems removed

2 tablespoons (28 ml) extra-virgin olive oil

1 teaspoon kosher salt

¼ teaspoon freshly ground black pepper

½ cup (120 ml) Creamy Roasted Garlic and Chive Dip (page 132)

2 avocados, peeled, pitted, and mashed

4 whole grain hamburger buns

½ cup (10 g) arugula

1 cup (240 g) fermented red cabbage kraut

1. Arrange a rack in the middle of the oven and preheat to 425°F (220°C, or gas mark 7).

2. Brush the mushrooms on both sides with oil and season with the salt and pepper. Place stem-side down on a rimmed baking sheet and roast for 15 minutes.

3. Once out of the oven, flip each mushroom cap over and spread an even layer of the Creamy Roasted Garlic and Chive Dip over the inside. To assemble, spread an even layer of the mashed avocado over the bottom of each bun. Top with the mushroom (spread-side up), followed by the arugula and kraut. Serve immediately.

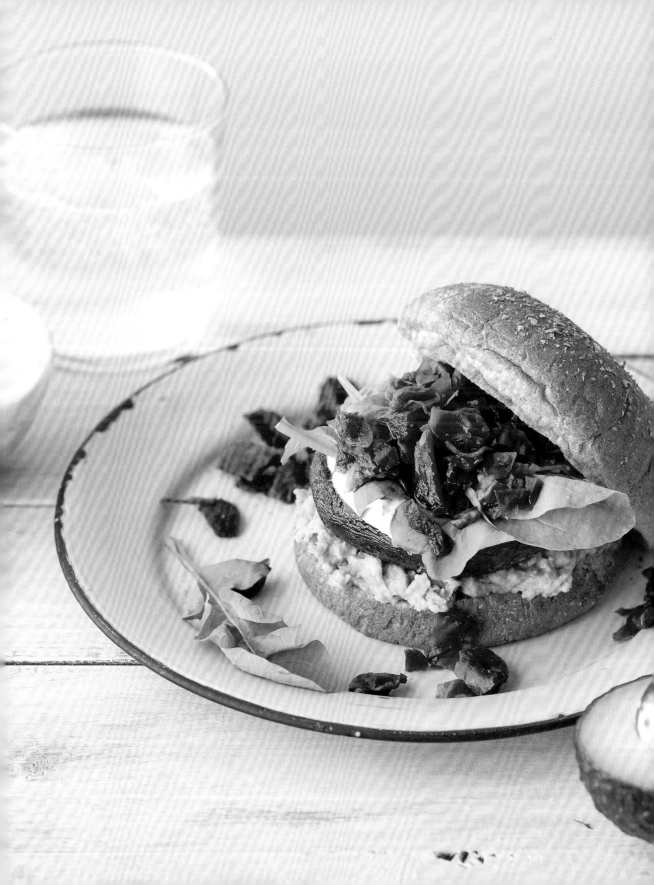

Tempeh Reuben

What this loaded sandwich, substantial enough for dinner, lacks in meat and traditional ingredients, it more than makes up for with big flavors and a whole lot of probiotics. It's inspired by a classic Reuben, but it swaps the corned beef for nutty tempeh and leans on gut-friendly foods like Greek yogurt, fermented pickles, and kraut.

SERVES 4

8 ounces (225 g) tempeh

3 tablespoons (45 ml) soy sauce
   or tamari

1 tablespoon (15 ml) Worcestershire
   sauce

1 clove garlic, minced

½ cup (115 g) live-culture plain
   Greek yogurt, preferably
   whole milk

2 tablespoons (30 g) ketchup

2 tablespoons (18 g) finely chopped
   fermented pickles

1 tablespoon (15 ml) extra-virgin
   olive oil

2 tablespoons (28 g) unsalted
   butter, room temperature

8 slices sourdough bread

1 cup (240 g) fermented sauerkraut

4 slices Swiss cheese

1. Slice the tempeh in half. Then, slice each half into quarters, making 8 thin pieces.

2. Whisk together the soy sauce, Worcestershire sauce, and garlic in a shallow container. Add the tempeh, gently mix to coat, and marinate for at least 30 minutes. Meanwhile, mix together the yogurt, ketchup, and pickles in a small bowl. Chill in the refrigerator.

3. Heat the oil in a large skillet over medium-high heat until shimmering. Add the tempeh and cook until golden brown, 2 minutes on each side.

4. To assemble the sandwiches, spread the butter on one side of each slice of bread. Flip and spread the yogurt dressing evenly over the opposite side. Divide the sauerkraut evenly among the spread side of 4 slices of the bread. Top each with a piece of the tempeh, followed by a slice of cheese, and finally the remaining slice of bread, spread-side down.

5. Heat a large frying pan or griddle over medium heat. Place the sandwiches in the pan and press down firmly with a metal spatula. Cook until the bottoms are golden brown, about 3 minutes. Carefully flip the sandwiches and cook for another 3 minutes on the opposite side.

6. Transfer the sandwiches to a cutting board. Slice them in half and serve immediately.

Creamy Mushroom Barley Risotto

Not only is barley a wholesome source of prebiotics, its toothsome texture and nutty taste make it a wonderful substitute for Arborio rice when preparing risotto. This lighter version skips the grated cheese in favor of protein-packed cultured cottage cheese, which makes this dish luxuriously creamy.

SERVES 4

4 cups (946 ml) low-sodium chicken or vegetable broth, warmed

3 tablespoons (45 ml) extra-virgin olive oil, divided

1 onion, diced

1 cup (200 g) pearl barley

1 teaspoon dried thyme

1¼ teaspoons kosher salt, divided

½ teaspoon freshly ground black pepper

½ cup (120 ml) dry white wine

8 ounces (225 g) assorted mushrooms, sliced

2 cloves garlic, minced

1 cup (225 g) cultured cottage cheese

1. Bring the broth to a gentle simmer in a medium saucepan.

2. Heat 1½ tablespoons (25 ml) of the oil in a large skillet over medium heat until shimmering. Add the onion and cook, stirring occasionally, until soft, about 5 minutes. Add the barley, thyme, 1 teaspoon of the salt, and the pepper, stir to coat with the oil, and cook until the barley is lightly toasted, about 3 minutes.

3. Stir in the wine and cook until the liquid is nearly absorbed. Add ½ cup (120 ml) of the broth and cook, stirring frequently, until most of the liquid has been absorbed. Continue adding the broth, ½ cup (120 ml) at a time, and after each addition, cook until most of the liquid has been absorbed. Continue until the barley is creamy and tender, with a slight bite.

4. Meanwhile, heat the remaining 1½ tablespoons (25 ml) of the oil in a separate skillet over medium-high heat until shimmering. Add the mushrooms and cook, stirring occasionally, until soft and crisp around the edges, about 10 minutes. Stir in the remaining ¼ teaspoon of salt and the garlic and cook 1 minute more.

5. Remove the barley from the heat and stir in the mushrooms and cottage cheese. Serve immediately.

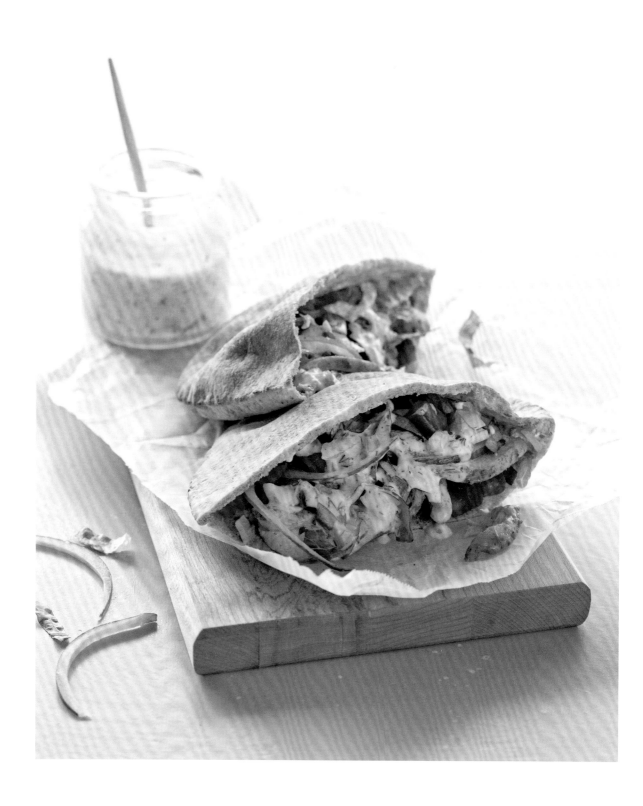

Chicken Shawarma Pockets *with* Probiotic Kefir Tzatziki

I have a confession: nearly every time I order shawarma, I'm really in it for the tzatziki. There is nothing quite as delicious as pairing this cool cucumber dip with smoky, spice-laden chicken. You'll want to marinate the chicken for at least an hour so it can soak up the flavors of the warm spices, though the more time, the better. I usually like to get a head start by making the tzatziki and soaking the chicken a day in advance.

SERVES 4

1 tablespoon (7 g) ground cumin

2 teaspoons sweet paprika

½ teaspoon ground turmeric

¼ teaspoon ground cinnamon

½ teaspoon kosher salt

½ teaspoon freshly ground black pepper

Pinch cayenne pepper

¼ cup (60 ml) extra-virgin olive oil

Juice of 2 lemons

2 pounds (900 g) boneless, skinless chicken thighs

4 whole wheat pitas, halved

1½ cups (71 g) chopped Romaine lettuce

1 plum tomato, chopped

½ small red onion, thinly sliced

1½ cups (355 ml) Probiotic Kefir Tzatziki (page 100)

1. Mix together the cumin, paprika, turmeric, cinnamon, salt, black pepper, and cayenne pepper in a large bowl. Add the olive oil and lemon juice and stir until all the spices are wet. Add the chicken and toss to fully coat with the spices. Cover and marinate in the refrigerator for at least 1 hour and up to overnight.

2. Arrange a rack in the middle of the oven and preheat to 425°F (220°C, or gas mark 7). Arrange the chicken in a single layer on a rimmed baking sheet. Cook until the chicken is lightly browned and cooked through, 20 to 25 minutes. Let cool.

3. Once the chicken is cool enough to handle, slice it into thin strips.

4. To serve, layer a spoonful of tzatziki at the bottom of each pita, followed by chicken, Romaine, tomatoes, red onion, and more tzatziki.

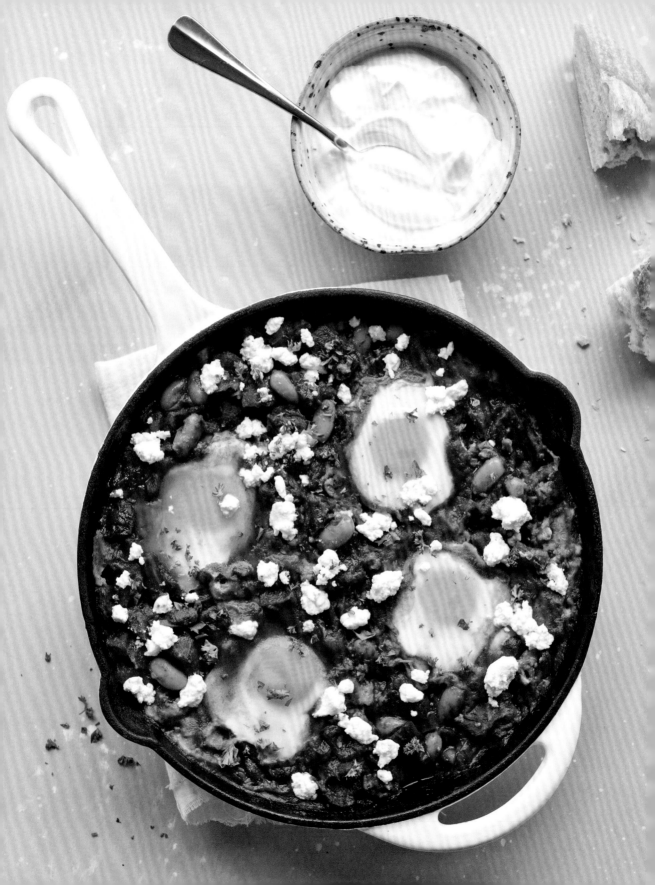

Easy White Bean Shakshuka

Shakshuka is the ultimate solution to eggs for dinner. Not only is it hearty and satisfying but it comes together surprisingly fast with a slew of pantry ingredients. A few generous dollops of Greek yogurt spooned over top just before serving is a quick and easy way to work some probiotics into a meal. Serve shakshuka with a few slices of good-quality sourdough on the side to dunk in the yolky eggs and mop up all the extra spiced-tomato sauce and yogurt.

SERVES 4

3 tablespoons (45 ml) extra-virgin olive oil

1 medium onion, diced

1 medium red bell pepper, chopped

3 cloves garlic, minced

1 teaspoon ground cumin

1 teaspoon sweet paprika

1¼ teaspoons kosher salt, divided

¼ teaspoon red pepper flakes

2 cans (15-ounce, or 425 g each) of cannellini beans, drained and rinsed

1 can (28-ounces, or 800 g) of fire-roasted diced tomatoes

6 large eggs

½ cup (115 g) live-culture plain Greek yogurt, preferably whole milk

4 slices sourdough bread, for serving

1. Heat the oil in a 12-inch (30 cm) skillet over medium heat until shimmering. Add the onion, bell pepper, garlic, cumin, paprika, 1 teaspoon of the salt, and the red pepper flakes and cook, stirring occasionally, until very soft, about 8 minutes. Stir in the beans and tomatoes and cook until the sauce thickens slightly, about 10 minutes.

2. Reduce the heat to low and use the back of a spoon to create small divots in the sauce. Gently crack the eggs into the skillet and sprinkle with the remaining ¼ teaspoon of salt. Cover and cook until the whites are set and the yolks are still runny, 6 to 8 minutes.

3. Divide the shakshuka among four plates, top with the yogurt, and serve with sourdough on the side.

Creamy Meyer Lemon Pasta *with* Basil

This seemingly summery pasta is fantastic to pull out in the middle of winter once Meyer lemons hit the market. Unlike regular lemons, these smooth-skinned, deep yellow citrus fruits have a mellower, sweeter taste that's noticeably less tart. The bright, creamy sauce is a breeze to mix together in a few minutes while the pasta is cooking. Stick with a twisted or tube pasta shape so the sauce has a chance to works its way into all the nooks and crannies.

SERVES 4

1 pound (455 g) dried fusilli, gemelli, or penne pasta

1½ cups (340 g) cultured cottage cheese

½ cup (50 g) finely grated Parmesan

Zest and juice of 2 Meyer lemons

¼ cup (10 g) roughly chopped fresh basil leaves

1 clove garlic, minced

½ teaspoon kosher salt

¼ teaspoon freshly ground black pepper

¼ teaspoon red pepper flakes

1. Bring a large pot of salted water to a boil and cook the pasta according to the package instructions until al dente. Drain well.

2. Meanwhile, add the cottage cheese, Parmesan, lemon zest and juice, basil, garlic, salt, black pepper, and red pepper flakes to a large bowl and stir well to combine.

3. Once the pasta is drained, add to the bowl with the cheese mixture and toss to coat. Serve immediately.

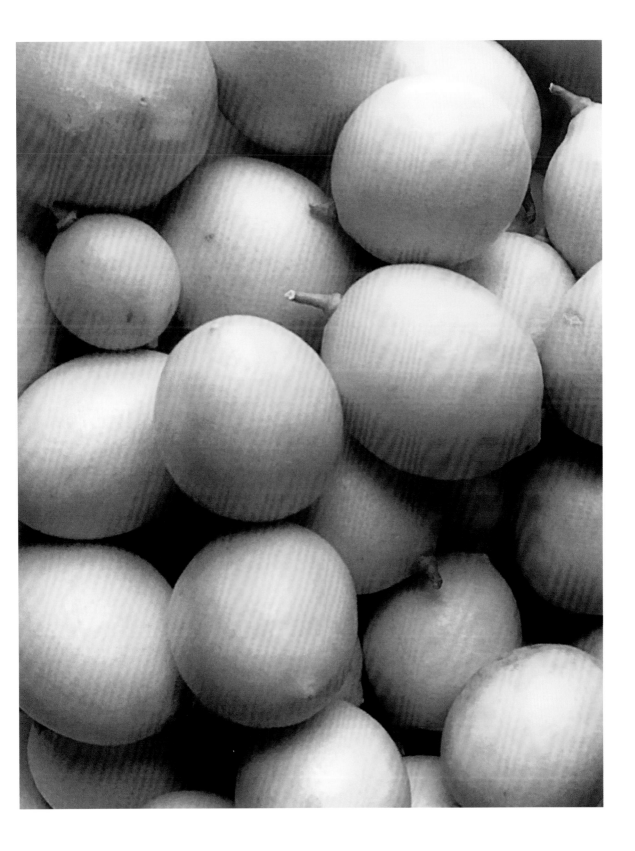

Cold Kimchi Soba Noodles

If you love a good noodle bowl, it's time to kick things up with some spicy kimchi. Rather than simply using it as a topping, you toss the kimchi with the noodles so the flavor has a chance to work its way through the whole bowl. But don't stop there. If you're lucky enough to have a jar with extra brine, I strongly recommend mixing some into the sauce for even more flavor.

SERVES 4

6 ounces (170 g) buckwheat soba noodles

2 tablespoons (28 cm) soy sauce or tamari

1 tablespoon (15 ml) rice vinegar

2 teaspoons kimchi brine (optional)

1 teaspoon toasted sesame oil

2 cups (140 g) thinly shredded red cabbage

1 cup (100 g) fermented kimchi, drained and chopped

3 scallions, thinly sliced

½ cup (8 g) finely chopped fresh cilantro leaves, plus more for topping

Red pepper flakes, for topping

1. Bring a large pot of salted water to a boil. Cook the soba noodles according to the package instructions. Drain the noodles and rinse thoroughly with cold water to remove the excess starch.

2. Meanwhile, whisk together the soy sauce, vinegar, kimchi brine (if using), and sesame oil in a large bowl. Add the soba noodles, red cabbage, kimchi, scallions, and cilantro. Toss well to combine. Divide the noodles among four bowls and then top with extra cilantro and red pepper flakes.

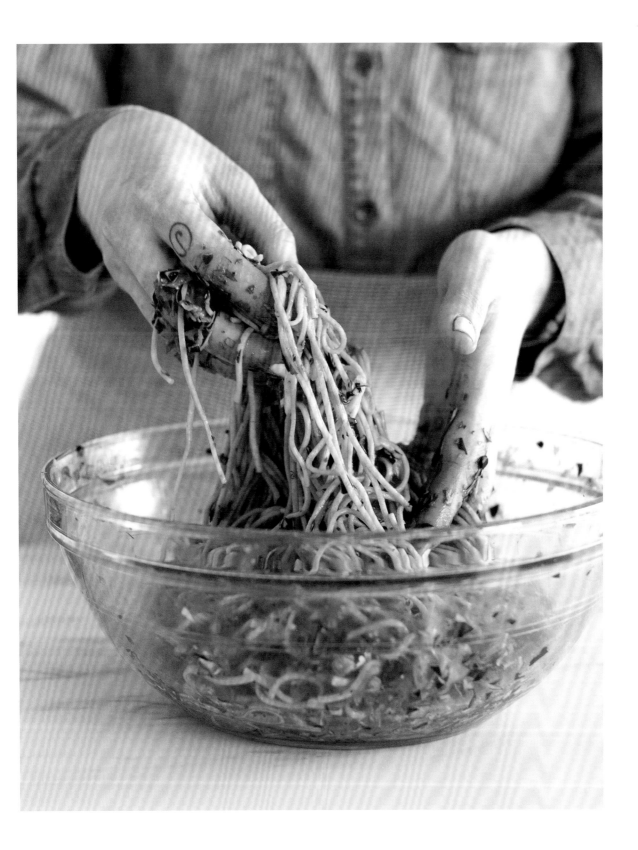

Cultured Macro Bowls

The thing I love most about macro bowls is knowing that I'm putting a truly balanced, healthy dinner on the table and putting something good into my body. Between the whole grains, legumes, fresh vegetables, fermented foods, and creamy toppings, there's just the right mix of carbs, protein, good fats, and gut-friendly ingredients. Plus, it also makes for an interesting mix of textures and flavors. Whether you opt for traditional sauerkraut or go for a version with a little more zip, you can't go wrong either way.

SERVES 4

4 large (or 6 medium) carrots, peeled and cut into ½-inch (1.3 cm) thick slices

1 tablespoon (15 ml) extra-virgin olive oil

1 teaspoon ground coriander

1 teaspoon kosher salt, divided

1 cup (173 g) quinoa, rinsed

¾ cup (144 g) brown lentils

2¾ cups (650 ml) water

2 cups (40 g) arugula

2 avocados, peeled, pitted, and thinly sliced

1 cup (240 g) fermented sauerkraut

1 cup (115 ml) live-culture plain Greek yogurt, preferably whole milk

Tahini, for drizzling

1. Arrange a rack in the middle of the oven and preheat to 400°F (200°C, or gas mark 6).

2. Add the carrots to a rimmed baking sheet. Drizzle with the oil and sprinkle with the coriander and ½ teaspoon of the salt. Toss to coat and spread in a single layer. Roast until tender, flipping once halfway through, about 20 minutes total.

3. Meanwhile, combine the quinoa, lentils, water, and the remaining ½ teaspoon of salt in a medium saucepan. Bring to a boil, then cover, reduce the heat to low, and simmer until tender, about 15 minutes. Remove from the heat, stir the mixture and then cover and let steam for 5 minutes.

4. To serve, divide the quinoa and lentils among four bowls. Top with the roasted carrots, arugula, avocado, kraut and yogurt and then finish with a drizzle of tahini.

Pasta *with*
Creamy Roasted Red Pepper Sauce

I'd like to clear the air about homemade pasta sauce being fussy and often time-consuming. Sure, it can be, but there are plenty of sauces that prove otherwise, including this one. It's a quick and easy no-cook sauce that gets whirled together in the food processor and can be ready before the pasta water even comes to a boil. While any kind of plain milk kefir will work here, whole milk kefir is the best choice, as it makes for a creamier sauce with more body.

SERVES 4

1 pound (455 g) tube-shaped pasta, such as penne or ziti

1 pound (455 g) roasted red peppers, drained

¾ cup (175 ml) live-culture plain milk kefir, preferably whole milk

½ cup (50 g) finely grated Parmesan, plus more for serving

3 cloves garlic

1 teaspoon sweet paprika

½ teaspoon kosher salt

¼ teaspoon freshly ground black pepper

Fresh basil leaves, for serving

1. Bring a large pot of salted water to a boil and cook the pasta according to the package instructions until al dente. Drain well.

2. Meanwhile, add the roasted red peppers, kefir, Parmesan, garlic, paprika, salt, and pepper to the bowl of a food processor or blender. Process continuously until well blended and mostly smooth.

3. Transfer the sauce to a large bowl. Add the drained, slightly cooled pasta and toss to coat. Divide among four bowls and top with fresh basil and more grated Parmesan.

Salmon Cakes with Quick Kimchi Aioli

A quick batch of salmon cakes is my number-one reason for keeping a few cans of wild salmon stashed in the pantry. They cook up with a crisp exterior and get a big boost of flavor, spice, and probiotics from creamy Quick Kimchi Aioli, which is mixed into the patties and used for dipping. Chilling the mixture adds some additional time to the prep, but it's worth it because it makes the cakes easier to form and helps them keep their shape when they hit the hot skillet.

SERVES 6

3 cans (6 ounces, or 170 g each) cans of wild salmon, drained

1 cup (235 ml) Quick Kimchi Aioli (page 99), divided

¼ cup (40 g) diced red onion

2 cloves garlic, minced

¼ cup (4 g) chopped fresh cilantro

1 large egg, beaten

½ teaspoon kosher salt

¼ teaspoon freshly ground black pepper

2 tablespoons (28 ml) extra-virgin olive oil

Kimchi, for topping (optional)

1. Add the salmon to a large bowl and use a fork to flake into small pieces. Add ¼ cup (60 ml) of the Quick Kimchi Aioli, the onion, garlic, cilantro, egg, salt, and pepper and mix well to combine. Cover and chill the mixture in the refrigerator for 10 minutes.

2. Shape the salmon mixture into 6 patties (about ½ cup [120 ml] and ½ inch [1.3 cm] thick). Place on a large plate or baking sheet and chill the patties in the refrigerator for 10 minutes.

3. Heat the oil in a large nonstick skillet over medium-high heat until shimmering. Add the salmon patties to the skillet, working in batches, if necessary. Cook until the bottom is lightly browned and crisp, about 4 minutes. Flip and cook the other side for another 4 minutes. Repeat with the remaining salmon patties.

4. Serve the salmon cakes with the remaining aioli and, if you like, extra kimchi.

Honey-Mustard Chicken Thighs

Sheet pan chicken thighs are a staple for my weeknight dinners (especially when I don't really feel like cooking) because they are so easy to pull off. The Creamy Honey-Mustard Dressing serves as both marinade and sauce. It starts with milk kefir, and, like yogurt, this probiotic-rich food keeps the chicken super tender and helps the thighs soak up the piquant flavors of the vinegar and mustard.

SERVES 4

2 pounds (900 g) boneless, skinless chicken thighs

¾ cup (175 ml) Creamy Honey-Mustard Dressing (page 94), divided

1. Combine the chicken thighs and ¼ cup (60 ml) of the Creamy Honey-Mustard Dressing in a shallow container and stir to coat. Cover and marinate in the refrigerator for at least 30 minutes and up to overnight.

2. Arrange a rack in the middle of the oven and preheat to 425°F (220°C, or gas mark 7).

3. Remove the chicken from the marinade, place on a rimmed baking sheet, and discard the remaining marinade. Roast until the chicken thighs are cooked through, 20 to 25 minutes.

4. To serve, drizzle the remaining dressing over the chicken thighs.

Try This Here

- Tangy Probiotic Potato Salad (page 177)
- Probiotic Miso-Tahini Slaw (page 176)
- Spring Vegetable Panzanella (page 128)

Mediterranean Stuffed Sweet Potatoes

Sweet potatoes rank high on my list of preferred foods for how amazingly versatile they are. Cook up a few during weekend meal prep, and you've got way more than a ready-made side dish. Stuffed with a slew of wholesome ingredients and finished with a drizzle of zingy, nutty sauce, this healthy, satisfying dinner is ready to please.

SERVES 4

½ cup (87 g) quinoa, rinsed

¾ cup (175 ml) water

1 teaspoon kosher salt, divided

2 tablespoons (28 ml) extra-virgin olive oil

½ small onion, diced

1 cup (240 g) chickpeas, drained and rinsed

¼ teaspoon red pepper flakes

4 cups (120 g) packed baby spinach

¼ cup (14 g) sundried tomatoes, chopped

3 cloves garlic, minced

Juice of 1 lemon

1 cup (235 ml) live-culture plain milk kefir, preferably whole milk

2 tablespoons (30 g) tahini

4 baked sweet potatoes, warmed

1. Combine the quinoa, water, and ½ teaspoon of the salt in a medium saucepan. Bring to a boil, then cover, reduce the heat to low, and simmer until tender, 12 to 15 minutes. Remove from the heat, stir the mixture, and then cover and let sit for 5 minutes.

2. Meanwhile, heat the oil in a large skillet over medium heat until shimmering. Add the onion, chickpeas, remaining ½ teaspoon salt, and red pepper flakes and cook, stirring occasionally, until the chickpeas are lightly browned, about 5 minutes. Add the spinach, sun-dried tomatoes, and garlic and cook, stirring occasionally, until the greens are wilted. Remove from the heat and stir in the quinoa and lemon juice.

3. Stir together the kefir and tahini in a small bowl.

4. To serve, split the sweet potatoes lengthwise down the center, pull open, and fluff the inside with a fork. Stuff the potato with the quinoa mixture and drizzle with kefir-tahini sauce.

Cider-Glazed Pork Tenderloin *with* Sauerkraut *and* Apples

Pork with apples and cabbage is a classic trio, and this recipe gives it a fun riff by swapping traditional braised cabbage leaves for fermented kraut. Red cabbage kraut adds a pop of color to the plate, though you really can't go wrong with any variety of fermented kraut here. It's worth adding a tiny pinch of cayenne pepper to the cider glaze. It's not spicy so much as it introduces the subtlest hint of heat to balance the sweetness of the apple and onion and the bite of the kraut.

SERVES 4

½ cup (120 ml) apple cider

2 tablespoons (28 ml) apple cider vinegar

1 tablespoon (15 g) whole grain mustard

Pinch cayenne pepper (optional)

1 pork tenderloin (1 to 1½-pounds, or 455 to 680 g)

1 tablespoon (15 ml) extra-virgin olive oil

1 tablespoon (14 g) unsalted butter

½ small onion, thinly sliced

1 apple, peeled and thinly sliced

½ teaspoon kosher salt, plus more for seasoning

¼ teaspoon freshly ground black pepper, plus more for seasoning

2 cups (480 g) fermented red cabbage kraut

1. Arrange a rack in the middle of the oven and preheat to 400°F (200°C, or gas mark 6).

2. Whisk together the apple cider, vinegar, mustard, and cayenne pepper (if using) in a small bowl. Set aside.

3. Pat the pork dry with paper towels and season generously all over with salt and pepper. Heat the oil in a large, oven-safe skillet over medium-high heat until shimmering. Add the pork to the skillet and sear on all sides until browned, about 8 minutes total. Transfer the skillet to the oven and cook for 12 to 14 minutes until the juices run clear.

4. Transfer the pork to a plate. Place the skillet over medium-high heat and melt the butter. Add the onion, apple, salt, and pepper and cook, stirring occasionally, for 5 minutes. Pour in the cider mixture and deglaze by using a wooden spoon to scrape any browned bits from the bottom of the pan. Bring to a boil and return the pork to the skillet. Cook, occasionally spooning the liquid over the pork, until the sauce is reduced by half, 2 to 3 minutes.

5. Slice the pork into medallions, spoon the cider glaze, apples, and onions over top, and serve with red cabbage kraut.

Farmers Market Pesto Pasta Salad

This is an ideal summer dinner in my book: a haul of farmers market veggies or the remnants of what I have in the crisper tossed with a big bowl of cooled pasta, plus a bright pesto and creamy cheese. Consider the vegetables listed in the recipe as a suggestion because just about anything you pick up at the market is fair game here, including bell peppers, corn, and carrots. I'd recommend sticking with the asparagus though, because, along with the Dandelion Pesto, it brings prebiotics to the table. And much as ricotta would, the farmer cheese adds a touch of creaminess (and probiotics) that makes the pasta even better.

SERVES 4 TO 6

1 pound (455 g) bowtie pasta

½ bundle thin asparagus, cut into 2-inch (5 cm) pieces

1 medium zucchini, chopped

1 cup (150 g) cherry tomatoes, halved

1 cup (75 g) chopped sugar snap peas

½ cup (120 ml) Dandelion Pesto (page 101)

1 cup (80 g) cultured farmer cheese

1. Bring a large pot of salted water to a boil and cook the pasta according to the package instructions until al dente. Drain well and cool completely.

2. Add the cooled pasta, asparagus, zucchini, tomatoes, peas, Dandelion Pesto, and farmer cheese to a large bowl and toss well to combine.

3. Serve chilled or at room temperature.

Miso Brown Rice *and* Tempeh Buddha Bowls

I have written a cookbook on Buddha bowls, so these one-bowl meals are near and dear to my heart and appear regularly in my dinner rotation. They're easy, satisfying, and delicious, and in this case, seamlessly work in a variety of probiotics, from super-savory miso paste (use any variety you have on hand) to tempeh, your favorite fermented kraut (or try swapping in lacto-fermented vegetables), and a generous drizzle of an herb-packed yogurt sauce.

SERVES 4

1 cup (190 g) brown rice

2 cups (475 ml) water

2 tablespoons (32 g) miso paste (any variety)

2 scallions, thinly sliced

2 medium sweet potatoes, peeled and cubed

2 tablespoons (28 ml) extra-virgin olive oil, divided

½ teaspoon kosher salt

¼ teaspoon freshly ground black pepper

8 ounces (225 g) tempeh, cut into thin strips

1 avocado, peeled, pitted, and chopped

1 cup (240 g) fermented sauer kraut

½ cup (120 ml) Herbed Yogurt Sauce (preferably made with cilantro) (page 96)

Toasted sesame seeds, for topping

1. Arrange a rack in the middle of the oven and preheat to 425°F (220° C, or gas mark 7).

2. Add the rice and water to a medium saucepan and bring to a boil. Reduce the heat to low, cover, and cook until the water is absorbed and the rice is tender, about 40 minutes. Remove from the heat and steam the rice with the lid on for 10 minutes. Add the miso paste and scallions and stir well to combine.

3. Meanwhile, add the sweet potatoes to a rimmed baking sheet, drizzle with 1 tablespoon (15 ml) of the oil, sprinkle with the salt and pepper, and toss to coat. Roast until tender and lightly browned, 20 to 25 minutes, flipping once halfway through.

4. Prepare the tempeh. Heat the remaining 1 tablespoon (15 ml) of oil in a large nonstick skillet over medium-high heat until shimmering. Add the tempeh strips and cook until golden brown all over, about 2 minutes per side.

5. To serve, divide the rice among four bowls and then top with sweet potatoes, tempeh, avocado, and kraut, drizzle with Herbed Yogurt Sauce, and garnish with toasted sesame seeds.

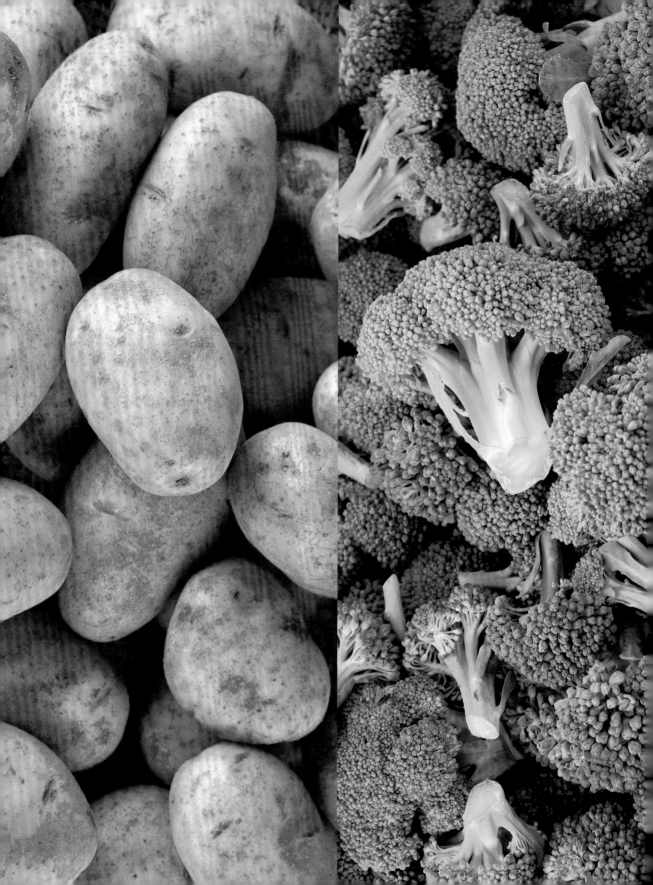

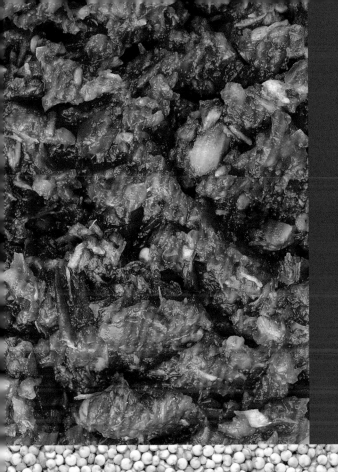

Sides

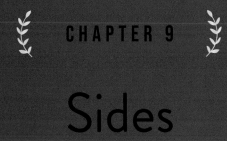

Miso-Butter Baked Potatoes

Don't be surprised if after dotting this humble side dish with a pat of miso butter your consumption of baked potatoes increases dramatically. That's precisely what happened to me. Mixed with softened butter, probiotic-rich miso paste adds a level of creaminess and deep savory flavor you just don't expect from a simple baked potato. It's a small upgrade that takes a potato from basic to brilliant.

SERVES 4

4 Russet potatoes, scrubbed

Extra-virgin olive oil

Kosher salt

4 tablespoons (55 g) unsalted butter, softened

2 tablespoons (32 g) white miso paste

2 scallions, thinly sliced, for topping

Flaky salt, for topping

1. Arrange a rack in the middle of the oven and preheat to 425°F (220°C, or gas mark 7).

2. Rub the potatoes all over with a thin layer of oil and sprinkle with kosher salt. Pierce the potato skin several times with a fork. Place the potatoes on a rimmed baking sheet and bake until the potatoes are tender and soft in the center with crisp skin, 45 to 60 minutes, depending on the size, flipping once halfway through.

3. Meanwhile, add the butter and miso paste to a small bowl and mix until well combined. Cover and store in the refrigerator until ready to serve.

4. To serve, split the potatoes down the center, fluff the flesh with a fork, and top with miso butter, sliced scallions, and flaky salt.

Haris Roasted Carrots *with* Cilantro-Yogurt Sauce

I've been making it for years and can easily say that this is one of my absolute best side dishes. Simply put, it has everything going for it. From an array of flavors that are sweet, a little spicy, fresh, and cool to the tender and crunchy textures you get with each bite, these carrots hit the spot every time and make an excellent partner to a huge variety of dinners.

Don't confuse young carrots with the stubby baby variety you buy for snacking. Young carrots, which sometimes have the leafy green stems still attached, have a tapered shape and concentrated sweet flavor, like their fully-grown counterparts.

SERVES 4

2 pounds (900 g) small young carrots, leafy tops trimmed

2 tablespoons (28 ml) extra-virgin olive oil

2 teaspoons harissa

½ teaspoon ground cumin

½ teaspoon kosher salt

¼ teaspoon freshly ground black pepper

½ cup (120 ml) Herbed Yogurt Sauce (made with cilantro) (page 96)

2 scallions, thinly sliced, for serving

Toasted pepitas, for serving

1. Arrange a rack in the middle of the oven and preheat to 425°F (220°C, or gas mark 7).

2. Add the carrots to a rimmed baking sheet, along with the oil, harissa, cumin, salt, and pepper and use your hands to toss to together. Arrange the carrots in a single layer. Roast until lightly browned and tender, about 25 minutes, tossing once halfway through.

3. To serve, add the carrots to a large plate, drizzle with the Herbed Yogurt Sauce, and sprinkle with sliced scallions and toasted pepitas.

What Is Harissa?

Harissa is a North African chili paste that's both smoky and spicy. It's important to note that not all brands of harissa are created equal, and a little can go a long way. While all are spicy, some are much more so than others. If you're new to cooking with this wonderful condiment or trying a new-to-you brand, give it a tiny taste before you start cooking. You can certainly increase or decrease the amount of harissa in the recipe to your spice preference.

Charred Broccoli *with* Miso-Tahini Sauce

Fans of classic roasted broccoli will love this stovetop side. Serving side dishes family style, with sauce layered on the bottom of the plate, is a small touch I think makes even the simplest dish feel a little more formal and reminiscent of something you'd get in a restaurant.

SERVES 4 TO 6

3 tablespoons (45 ml) extra-virgin olive oil

1 large head broccoli, cut into bite-size florets

½ teaspoon kosher salt

¼ teaspoon red pepper flakes

2 cloves garlic, chopped

Juice of ½ lemon

¼ cup (60 ml) Miso-Tahini Sauce (page 97)

¼ cup (25 g) toasted almonds, chopped

1. Heat the oil in a large cast-iron skillet over medium-high heat until shimmering. Add the broccoli, salt, and red pepper flakes. Toss to coat with the oil and spread in a single layer. Cook undisturbed until the bottoms of the florets are well browned, about 4 minutes. Flip and char the other side, about 4 minutes more.

2. Add the garlic and cook, stirring occasionally, for 1 minute more. Remove the pan from the heat and squeeze the juice from the lemon over top.

3. To serve, spread the Miso-Tahini Sauce in an even layer on a large plate or platter. Top with the broccoli and sprinkle with the almonds.

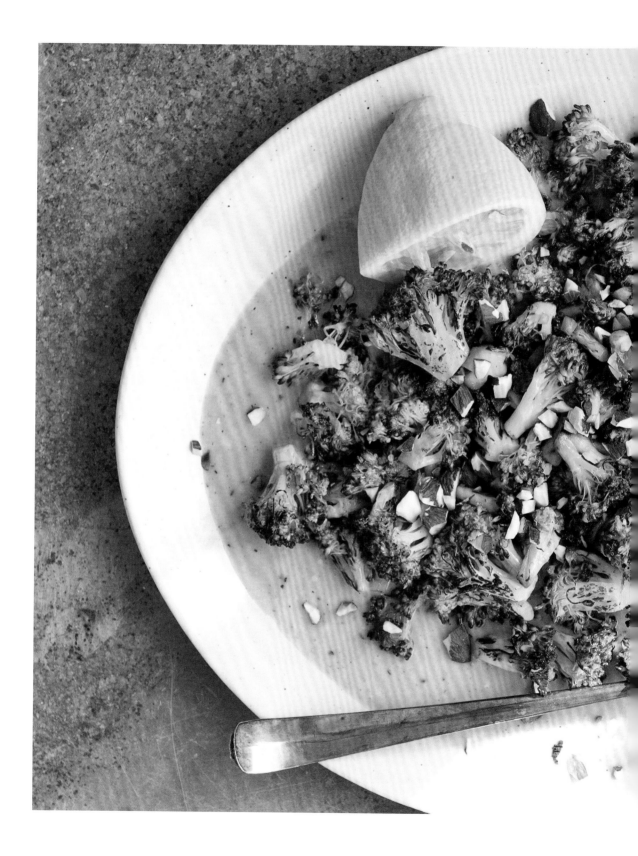

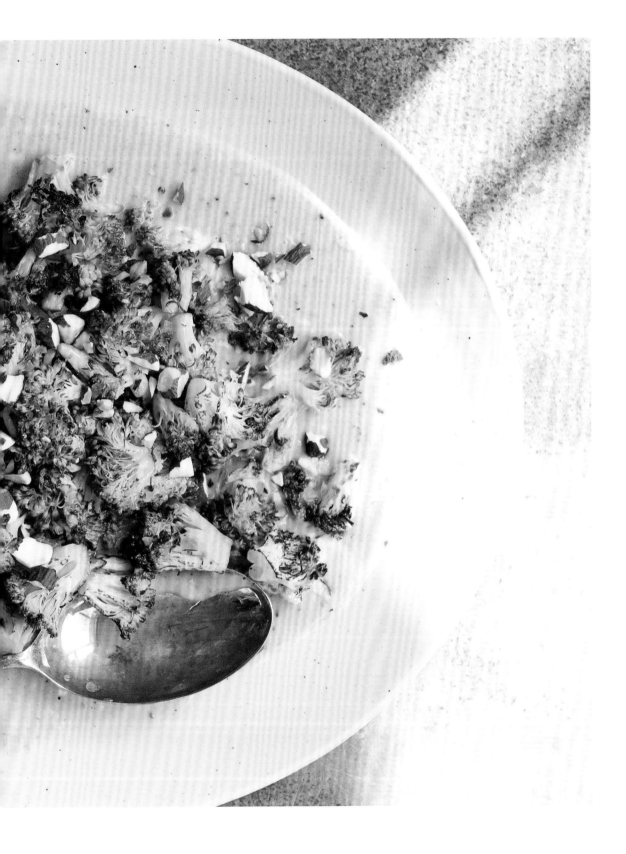

Quick Sugar Snap Peas *with* Orange-Miso Vinaigrette

Let me introduce you to a fantastic way to eat snap peas—cooked for just a couple minutes in a pot of salty, boiling water and then tossed with a simple vinaigrette. The citrus dressing is a bright and refreshing partner to snap peas and pairs well with just about anything you're cooking. The snap peas can be blanched a day in advance and stored in the refrigerator until you're ready to serve.

SERVES 4

Kosher salt

1 pound (455 g) sugar snap peas, trimmed

⅓ cup (80 ml) Orange-Miso Vinaigrette (page 92)

1 shallot, minced

¼ cup (4 g) fresh chopped cilantro

1 teaspoon toasted sesame seeds, plus more for garnish

1. Bring a large pot of salted water to a boil. Add the snap peas and cook until just barely tender but still crisp, about 2 minutes. Drain and transfer to an ice bath.

2. Whisk together the Orange-Miso Vinaigrette, shallot, cilantro, and sesame seeds in a large bowl. Drain the snap peas, add them to the bowl with the vinaigrette, and mix.

3. Serve the snap peas at room temperature and top with additional sesame seeds, if desired.

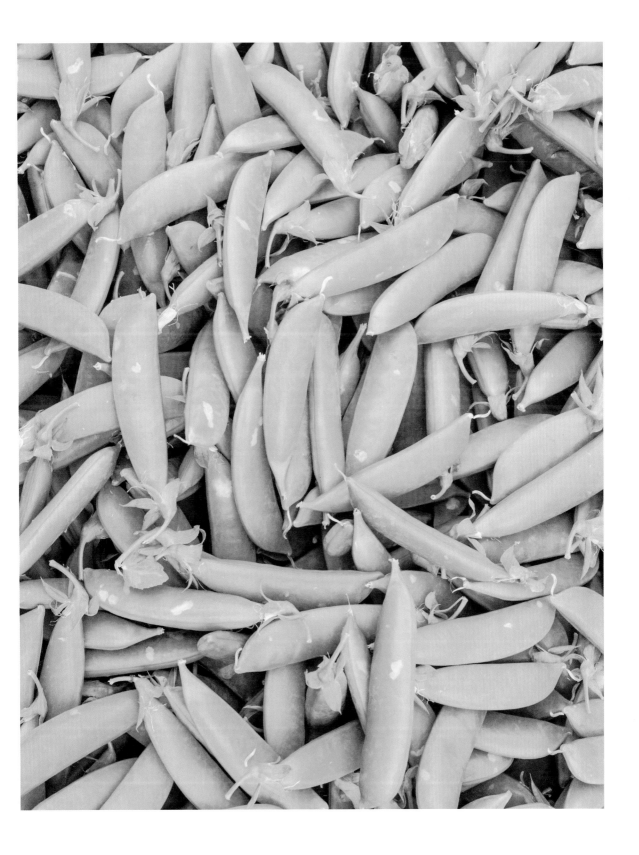

Probiotic Miso-Tahini Slaw

I love vibrant, crunchy slaws. They're a go-to especially anytime I need to pull together a side dish in a hurry. And one of my favorite tricks for adding even more flavor (and gut-friendly benefits) without any extra work is mixing in whatever kind of fermented kraut I have lingering in the fridge. While you can certainly prep the vegetables on your own, don't overlook the convenience of starting with a couple of bags of preshredded slaw, so all that's left to do is whisk together the dressing.

SERVES 4 TO 6

¾ cup (175 ml) Miso-Tahini Sauce, divided (page 97)

2 cups (140 g) thinly shredded red cabbage

10 ounces (280 g) broccoli slaw

4 scallions, thinly sliced

1 cup (240 g) fermented sauerkraut

½ cup (46 g) toasted sliced almonds

1. Add ½ cup (120 ml) of the Miso-Tahini Sauce to a large bowl, along with the cabbage, broccoli slaw, scallions, and sauerkraut. Toss well to combine.

2. Mix with additional sauce, if desired. Top with almonds and serve the slaw chilled or at room temperature.

Tangy Probiotic Potato Salad

Here, milk kefir takes the place of typical potato salad mix-ins, such as sour cream or mayonnaise. Not only does it give this timeless side a dose of probiotics, but combined with a splash of apple cider vinegar, it also makes for a light and lively dressing that really jazzes up the potatoes. While the potato salad can certainly be served immediately after it's prepared, it gets better as it sits, giving the potatoes plenty of time to soak up the punchy dressing. With that in mind, try making it a day in advance if you have the time.

SERVES 6

2 pounds (900 g) baby purple, red, or new potatoes, or a combination of all three

1 tablespoon (15 g) plus ¼ teaspoon kosher salt, divided

⅔ cup (160 ml) live-culture plain milk kefir, preferably whole milk

2 tablespoons (28 ml) apple cider vinegar

2 teaspoons Dijon mustard

½ teaspoon freshly ground black pepper

⅓ cup (33 g) thinly sliced scallions

1 large celery rib, diced

1. Place the potatoes in a large saucepan, cover with cold water, and add 1 tablespoon (15 g) of the salt. Bring to a boil and then reduce the heat to a simmer and cook the potatoes until tender, 10 to 12 minutes. Drain the potatoes and cool completely. Once cool, halve the potatoes or quarter them if using larger potatoes.

2. Meanwhile, whisk together the kefir, vinegar, mustard, pepper, and remaining ¼ teaspoon of salt in a large bowl. Stir in the scallions and celery. Add the potatoes and stir to combine.

3. Cover and refrigerate the salad until ready to serve.

Creamy Cucumber Salad

It is impossible to think about cucumber salad without immediately envisioning summertime. Don't you agree? It's a quintessential summer side—though I've taken to tossing it together all year long—and this version gets added probiotics thanks to milk kefir and prebiotics from raw onion and garlic. I recommend using whole milk kefir for an extra-creamy dressing.

SERVES 4 TO 6

1 cup (235 ml) live-culture plain milk kefir, preferably whole milk

2 tablespoons (28 ml) apple cider vinegar

1 tablespoon (15 ml) extra-virgin olive oil

¼ cup (16 g) chopped fresh dill

1 small clove garlic, minced

½ teaspoon kosher salt

¼ teaspoon freshly ground black pepper

2 large cucumbers, peeled and thinly sliced into rounds

½ small red onion, halved and thinly sliced

1. Mix together the kefir, vinegar, oil, dill, garlic, salt, and pepper in a large bowl.

2. Add the cucumbers and red onion and stir well to coat. Cover and refrigerate the salad for 30 minutes before serving.

Quick Miso Quinoa

As so many good recipes do, this one started a long time ago by pulling bits and bobs of ingredients from the pantry and refrigerator in an effort to scrape together a last-minute side dish—something more than a basic pot of plain quinoa. The result was surprisingly delightful. Over time, I've tweaked it by toasting the quinoa in a splash of coconut oil for an extra-nutty undertone, upping the amount of savory miso, and including scallions for a little added probiotic and prebiotic benefit. This dish is meant to be easy and versatile, so any kind of miso paste you have handy will work, with white miso lending a mellower flavor and red miso adding a deeper, nuttier taste.

SERVES 4

1 tablespoon (14 g) coconut oil

1 cup (173 g) quinoa, rinsed

1¾ cups (410 ml) low-sodium chicken broth, vegetable broth, or water

½ teaspoon kosher salt

1 tablespoon (16 g) miso paste, any variety

1 tablespoon (15 ml) soy sauce or tamari

2 teaspoons rice vinegar

3 scallions, thinly sliced

1. Heat the coconut oil in a medium saucepan over medium heat until shimmering. Add the quinoa and toast, stirring occasionally, for 3 minutes.

2. Slowly pour in the broth or water and salt. Bring to a boil, then cover, reduce the heat to low, and simmer until tender, about 15 minutes. Remove from the heat, stir the mixture, and then cool for 5 minutes.

3. Add the miso paste, soy sauce, vinegar, and scallions, stir well with a fork to combine, and serve.

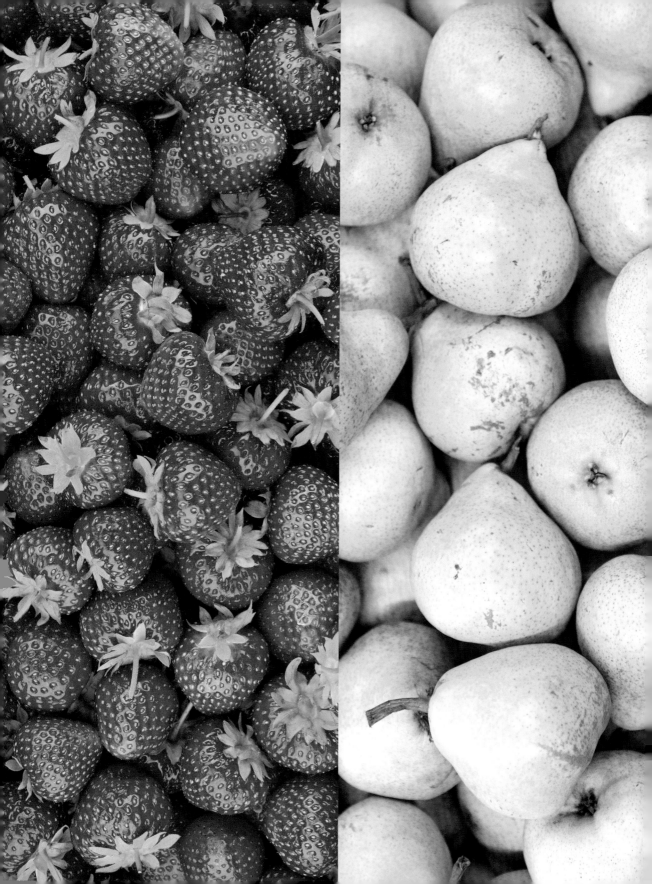

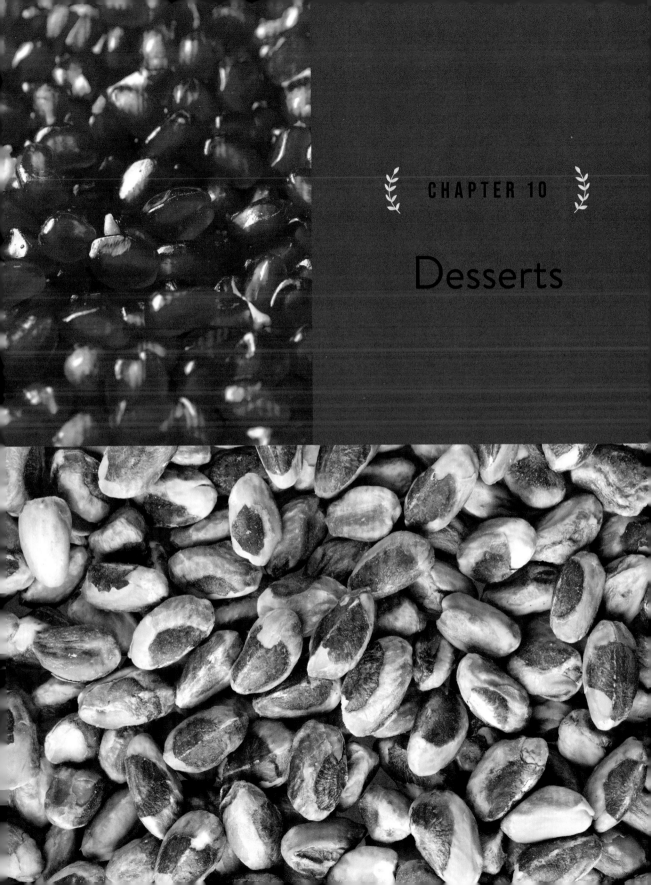

Desserts

Fruit Salad *with* Kefir Dressing

About a year ago, I dressed a simple fruit salad with vinaigrette for the first time and I couldn't believe I hadn't been doing it forever. It's the instant upgrade that will transform even the most basic bowl of fruit into one that feels gourmet. It's also a great touch when you're working with berries that aren't quite ripe enough.

SERVES 6

3 cups (456 g) chopped pineapple

2 cups (300 g) red grapes, halved

½ pint (175 g) strawberries, stems removed and quartered

1 heaping cup (145 g) blueberries

1 heaping cup (125 g) raspberries

1 tablespoon (6 g) chopped fresh mint

⅓ cup (80 ml) Creamy Kefir Poppy Seed Dressing (page 90)

1. Place the pineapple, grapes, strawberries, blueberries, raspberries, and mint in a large bowl and toss gently to combine.

2. Just before serving, pour the Creamy Kefir Poppy Seed Dressing over the fruit salad and toss gently to coat, being careful not to crush the berries.

Kombucha Floats

While it's been years since I've had them, ice cream sodas and floats were some of my favorite desserts as a kid. I loved the way the ice cream melted into the soda, giving it a mellow creaminess to balance the stinging carbonation, and the little crystals that formed around the scoop of ice cream. Guess what—kombucha works the exact same way! This is my version of a grown-up float. It works with both ice cream and sorbet, and any flavor of kombucha is fair game, so get creative with your combinations.

SERVES 2

4 scoops ice cream or sorbet of choice

16 ounces (475 ml) kombucha

1. Divide the ice cream or sorbet between two chilled glasses. I like to use the tall, soda-fountain variety.

2. Pour the kombucha over top. Be sure to pour slowly, so the carbonation doesn't cause a spillover. Serve the sweet treat immediately with a straw and a spoon and enjoy!

Popular Flavor Combinations

- *Vanilla Ice Cream + Pomegranate Kombucha*
- *Raspberry Sorbet + Original Kombucha*
- *Blackberry Sorbet + Lavender Kombucha*
- *Blood Orange Sorbet + Ginger Kombucha*

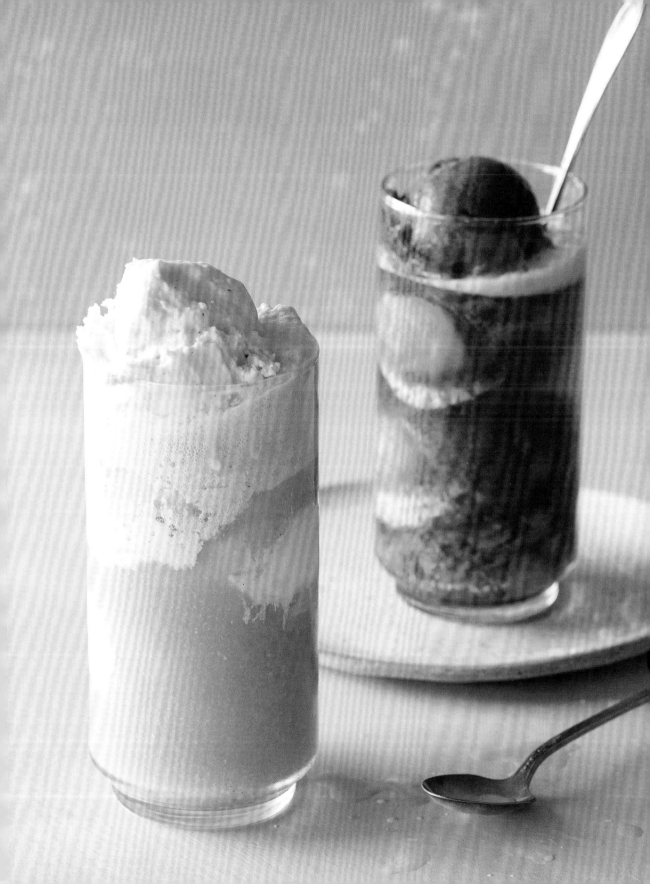

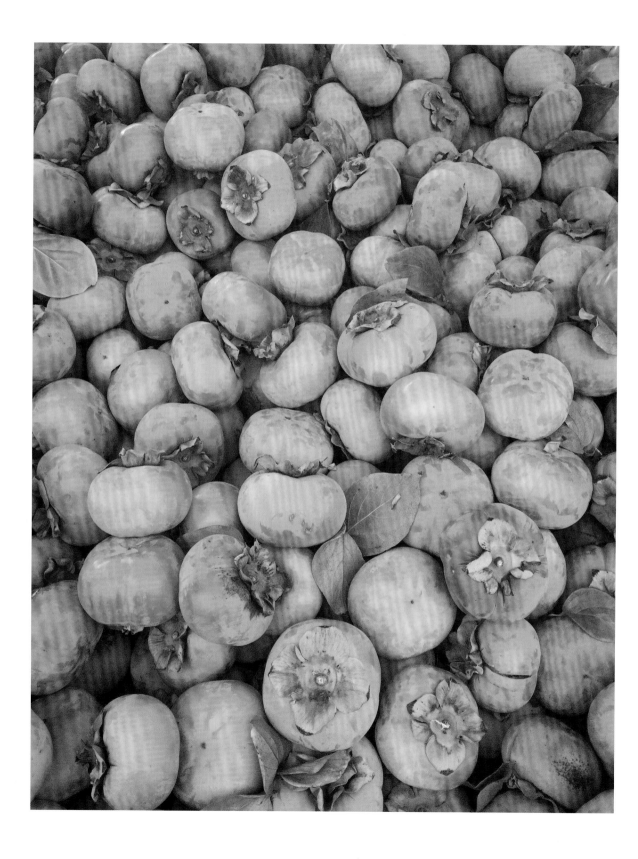

Whipped Yogurt *with* Roasted Persimmons

I eat yogurt so often for breakfast that I never considered it for dessert, until now. The trick is whipping it along with a splash of cream. It's magical! Try it once, and I promise, you'll never look back. Light and airy whipped yogurt satisfies my dessert craving without loading up on sugar or being too rich. It's quick and easy enough to pull off on a weeknight, yet special enough to serve when you have friends over for dinner.

SERVES 4

2 Fuyu persimmons

1 tablespoon (15 ml) extra-virgin olive oil

¼ teaspoon ground cardamom

Pinch kosher salt

1 cup (115 ml) live-culture plain Greek yogurt, preferably whole milk

½ cup (120 ml) heavy cream

1 tablespoon (13 g) granulated sugar

¼ cup (44 g) pomegranate arils

¼ cup (31 g) toasted pistachios, chopped

1. Preheat the oven to 425°F (220°C, or gas mark 7).

2. Trim the persimmons and cut each fruit into 6 wedges. Toss with the oil, cardamom, and salt. Spread in a single layer in a cast-iron skillet. Roast until tender and lightly caramelized, about 15 minutes.

3. Meanwhile, add the yogurt, cream, and sugar to a large bowl and beat with an electric mixer on high speed (or in a stand mixer with the whisk attachment) until stiff peaks form, about 2 minutes.

4. Divide the yogurt among four bowls, top with the roasted persimmons, pomegranate arils, and pistachios.

Strawberry Yogurt Ice Pops

These healthy yogurt pops are an amazing summer treat in part because, well, they simply taste like summer, but also because they couldn't be easier to pull off. Save these pops for when you have a container of ripe, juicy berries—the flavor will be all the better for it.

MAKES 10 ICE POPS

1 pound (455 g) strawberries, stems removed and roughly chopped

1½ cups (355 ml) live-culture plain Greek yogurt, preferably whole milk

¼ cup (85 g) honey, preferably raw

1 tablespoon (15 ml) freshly squeezed lemon juice

Pinch kosher salt

1. Place all the ingredients in a blender or food processor and process continuously until smooth, 1 to 2 minutes.

2. Divide the mixture among ice pop molds, insert a stick, if necessary, and freeze for at least 6 hours.

3. To unmold, run the ice pops under hot water for a few seconds and the mold will easily slide off.

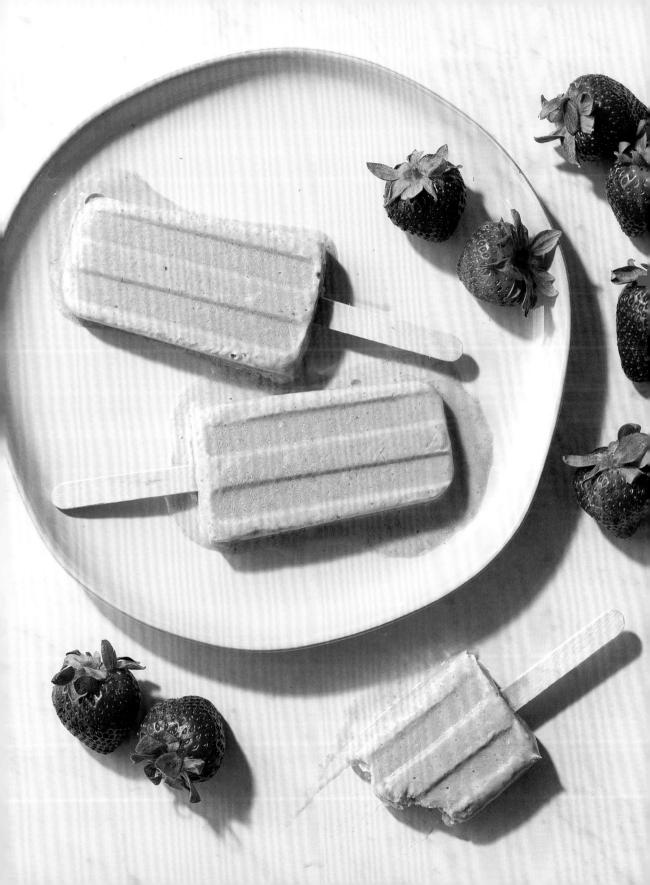

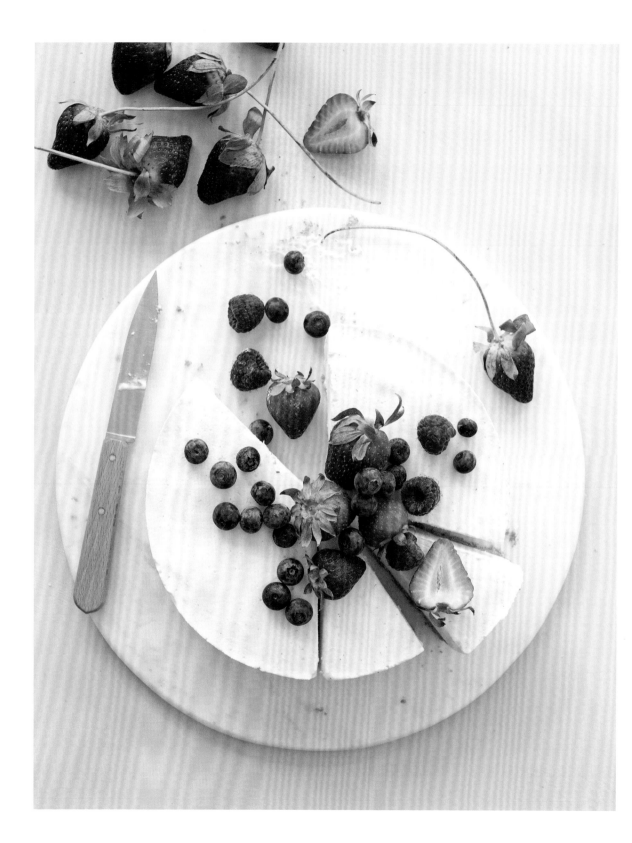

No-Bake Vanilla Bean Cheesecake

While I was growing up, my mom made a fruit-topped no-bake cream cheese pie that was always one of the highlights of my summer. Inspired by her rich and creamy dessert, this version comes with a much lighter twist that cuts back on the sugar and swaps the cream cheese for gut-friendly cultured cottage cheese. When whipped in the food processor, the small curds of this probiotic-rich cottage cheese are transformed into a smooth, creamy, and slightly dense texture. You'll want to plan ahead, as the cheesecake benefits from chilling in the refrigerator for at least eight hours to firm up nicely.

SERVES 8 TO 12

FOR THE CRUST:

9 full-size graham crackers (or 1¼ cup [150 g] graham cracker crumbs)

1 tablespoon (13 g) granulated sugar

4 tablespoons (55 g) unsalted butter, melted and slightly cooled

FOR THE FILLING:

16 ounces (455 g) cultured cottage cheese

1 vanilla bean

¼ cup (50 g) granulated sugar

¼ teaspoon kosher salt

1 cup (235 ml) heavy cream

1. To make the crust, add the graham crackers and sugar to a food processor and process continuously until an even crumb forms. Slowly pour in the butter and pulse to combine. Transfer the graham cracker crumbs to an 8-inch (20 cm) springform pan. Firmly press the crumbs in an even layer to the edges of the pan, using your fingers. Refrigerate the crust while you prepare the filling.

2. Wipe out the food processor bowl and blade. Add the cottage cheese to the food processor. Split the vanilla bean in half lengthwise with a paring knife. Use the tip of the knife to scrape the vanilla bean seeds from the pod and add to the cottage cheese. Process continuously for 30 seconds. With the machine running, slowly pour in the sugar and salt and continue to blend until smooth, about 30 seconds more.

3. Add the cream to a large bowl and beat with a hand mixer at high speed until stiff peaks form. Alternatively, use a stand mixer fitted with the whisk attachment. Gently fold the cottage cheese mixture into the whipped cream.

4. Transfer the filling to the prepared pan and spread in an even layer over the graham cracker crust.

5. Cover and refrigerate for at least 8 hours before slicing and serving.

Strawberry-Basil Kombucha Granita

A granita is basically a high-brow slushy, with a dry, flaky texture. While it does take some time to make, it's extremely low effort and really couldn't be easier. The kombucha loses some of its fizz once frozen, though plenty of its fruit flavor and a subtle hint of fresh herbs still come through in the granita. If you don't have basil handy, fresh mint makes a nice substitute in this dessert.

SERVES 4

⅓ cup (80 ml) water

¼ cup (50 g) granulated sugar

½ cup (12 g) packed rubbed and torn fresh basil leaves or mint leaves (See Cooking Tip! below.)

16 ounces (475 ml) strawberry kombucha

1. Combine the water and sugar in a small saucepan. Bring to a boil and then cook, stirring until the sugar is dissolved. Remove from the heat, stir in the basil or mint leaves, and cool completely.

2. Once cool, strain and press the simple syrup from the basil leaves and discard the leaves. Add the simple syrup and kombucha to an 8 × 8-inch (20 × 20 cm) baking pan or similar-size dish and stir to combine.

3. Freeze for 30 minutes. Remove the pan from the freezer and gently scrape the mixture with a fork to break it up into frozen bits. Return to the freezer. Repeat this process every 30 minutes until the granita has a dry, flaky texture, no longer clumps together, and is completely frozen, about 2 hours.

Cooking Tip!

Here are a couple of small tricks to help you maximize the flavor from fresh basil leaves. First, you'll want to rub and tear the herb leaves before adding them to the simple syrup—this will help release more of the basil's natural oils, which is where the flavor lives. Second, when straining the leaves from the simple syrup, use a fork to press them into the strainer to eke out an extra burst of flavor.

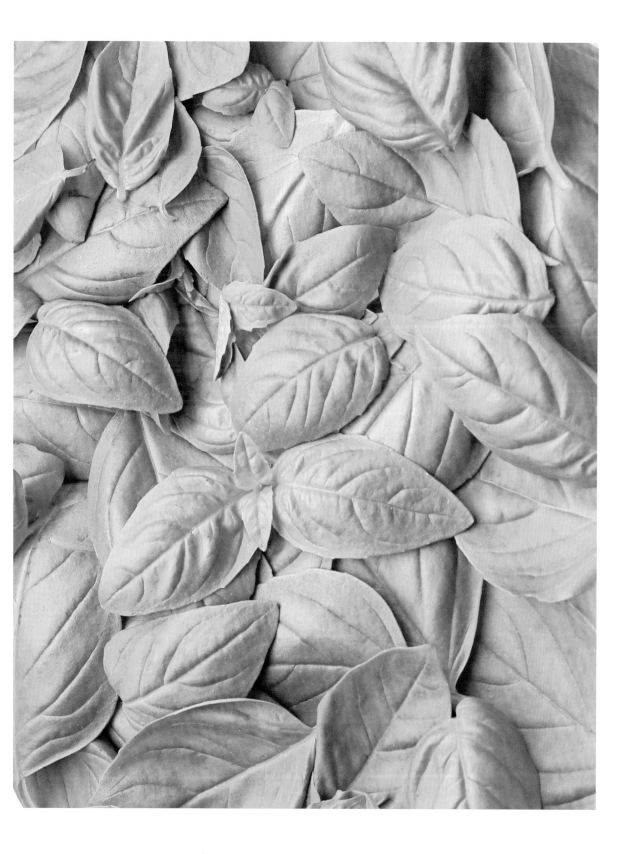

Coconut-Lime Kefir Ice Pops

Coconut and lime is a delightful flavor combination for ice pops. Come the middle of summer when it feels like it couldn't possibly get any hotter, these pops are so refreshing. And on the flip side, when the snow is piled high, this tropical-inspired duo fuels a daydream of sun and sand. Creamy whole milk kefir lends even more flavor to these cool and refreshing pops, and the tartness of the lime juice balances the richness of the coconut milk.

MAKES 10 ICE POPS

1 can (14 ounces, or 415 ml) of unsweetened coconut milk

¾ cup (175 ml) live-culture plain kefir, preferably whole milk

¼ cup (85 g) honey, preferably raw

Juice of 2 limes

Zest of 1 lime

½ cup (40 g) unsweetened shredded coconut (optional)

Pinch kosher salt

1. Place all the ingredients in a blender or food processor and process continuously until smooth, about 1 minute.

2. Divide the mixture among ice pop molds, insert a stick, if necessary, and freeze for at least 6 hours.

3. To unmold, run the ice pops under hot water for a few seconds and the mold will easily slide off.

Caramelized Pears with Maple Yogurt

This cinnamon-scented dessert will likely remind you a little of apple pie. That's exactly where the inspiration came from, though this version puts pears squarely in the spotlight. If you have pears that aren't ripe yet, the heat of the skillet is just the thing to soften them up and make them perfect for eating. But what really makes this sweet treat sing is the maple yogurt at the bottom of the bowl.

SERVES 4

1 cup (115 g) live-culture plain Greek yogurt, preferably whole milk

2 tablespoons (28 ml) pure maple syrup

1½ teaspoons (28 g) vanilla extract, divided

2 tablespoons unsalted butter

2 Anjou or Bartlett pears, peeled and quartered

3 tablespoons (45 g) light brown sugar

Pinch kosher salt

2 tablespoons (28 ml) water

2 tablespoons (12 g) sliced toasted almonds

Ground cinnamon, for serving

1. Mix together the yogurt, maple syrup, and ½ teaspoon of the vanilla in a small bowl. Set aside.

2. Melt the butter in a large skillet over medium heat. Add the pears, cut-side down at first, and cook, flipping them occasionally, until golden brown, 3 to 5 minutes. Add the sugar and salt to the skillet, stir to coat the pears, and cook, swirling the pan occasionally, for 5 minutes more. Add the water and the remaining 1 teaspoon of vanilla and swirl the pan to release the caramel from the bottom.

3. To serve, divide the yogurt among four bowls and then top with the pears, sliced almonds, and a sprinkle of cinnamon.

Mango Frozen Yogurt Nice Cream

If you're like me and you want instant-gratification desserts without having to wait for frozen yogurt or ice cream to harden after churning, you're going to love this fruity, no-churn treat. About five minutes stand between you and this healthy frozen yogurt. It's at its best soon after it's blitzed together, when it has the consistency of thick and creamy soft serve. If you choose to stash it in the freezer, plan to let it sit at room temperature to soften slightly and become scoopable before serving. Use whole milk yogurt for the creamiest dessert.

SERVES 2 TO 4

2 heaping cups (350 g) frozen mango chunks

1 cup (115 g) live-culture plain Greek yogurt, preferably whole milk

1 teaspoon granulated sugar

1 teaspoon pure vanilla extract

Pinch kosher salt

1. Add the mango to a food processor and process continuously until crumbly. Scrape down the sides of the bowl and then add the yogurt, sugar, vanilla, and salt. Process continuously until smooth and creamy, about 2 minutes.

2. Serve the nice cream immediately for a soft-serve consistency or for a firmer texture, transfer to a lidded, airtight container and freeze for at least 2 hours.

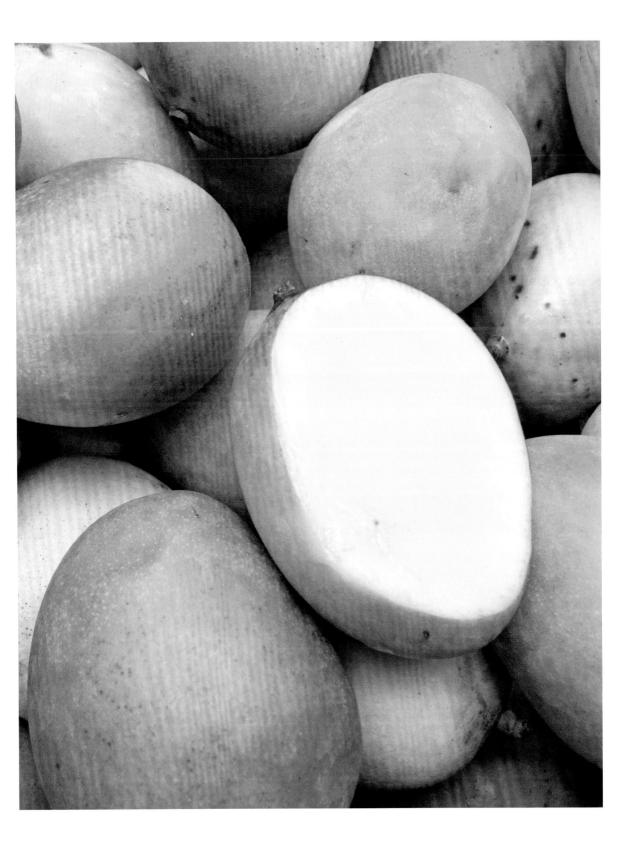

Resources

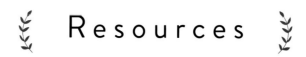

Books

Challa, Shekhar. *Probiotics for Dummies*. Wiley, 2012.

Hattner, Jo Ann and Anderes, Susan. *Gut Insight*. Hattner Nutrition, 2009.

Huffnagle, Gary B. and Wernick, Sarah. *The Probiotics Revolution*. Bantam Books, 2008.

Katz, Sandor Ellix. *The Art of Fermentation*. Chelsea Green Publishing, 2012.

Mayer, Emeran. *The Mind-Gut Connection*. Harper Wave, 2018.

Smolyansky, Julie. *The Kefir Cookbook*. HarperOne, 2018.

Sonnenburg, Justin and Sonnenburg, Erica. *The Good Gut*. Penguin Books, 2016.

Tannis, Allison. *Probiotic Rescue*. Wiley, 2008.

Institutions and Organizations

Gut Microbiota for Health
www.gutmicrobiotaforhealth.com

Mayo Clinic
www.mayoclinic.org

National Institutes of Health
www.nih.gov

National Center for Complementary and Integrative Health
nccih.nih.gov

PRODUCTS

Cottage Cheese and Kefir

Good Culture
www.goodculture.com

Horizon Organic
www.horizon.com

Nancy's
www.nancysyogurt.com

Lifeway
www.lifewaykefir.com

Yogurt and Skyr

Fage
www.usa.fage

Stonyfield
www.stonyfield.com

Anita's
www.anitas.com

The Coconut Cult
www.thecoconutcult.com

COYO
www.coyo.com

Icelandic Provisions
www.icelandicprovisions.com

Siggi's
www.siggis.com

Fermented Foods

Bubbies
www.bubbies.com

The Brinery
www.thebrinery.com

Hawthorne Valley
ferments.hawthornevalley.org

Ozuké
www.ozuke.com

Mother In Law's
www.milkimchi.com

Sunja's
www.sunjaskimchi.com

Miso Master
www.great-eastern-sun.com/product-category/miso-master-miso

Kombucha

GT's Living Foods
www.gtslivingfoods.com

Health-Ade
www.health-ade.com

Acknowledgments

First and foremost, a big thank you to the entire team at Harvard Common Press and Quarto for their work in bringing this book to life. To my editor, Dan Rosenberg, for coaching me along, showing me that I'm capable of big things in a short amount of time, and his continued support. Thank you also to Renae Haines for her behind the scenes work in moving this project along and Marissa Giambrone for making this book so beautiful.

Many thanks to Maria Siriano for once again capturing my vision so wonderfully and making the food look so delectable.

The Kitchn team. You all constantly inspire me and make me a better writer and person.

My gratitude to my family and friends for all your feedback throughout the process of creating and developing this book. Your endless support, love, encouragement, and willingness to taste and test my recipes means the world to me. I could not have done this without you.

And finally, the biggest and most heartfelt thank you to my husband, Lucien. You have been my dishwasher, taste tester, and number one supporter every step of the way. Thank you for always believing in me and pushing me to follow my dreams.

About the Author

Kelli Foster is the author of *Buddha Bowls* and *Everyday Freekeh Meals* as well as a food editor at the popular cooking site The Kitchn. Her work has also been featured on Greatist and *The Dr. Oz Show*. She lives in New York City.

Index